DASH & Mediterranean Diets Guide

By

Stephanie N. Collins

Legal & Disclaimer

The information contained in this book is not designed to replace or take the place of any form of medicine or professional medical advice. The information in this book has been provided for educational and entertainment purposes only.

The information contained in this book has been compiled from sources deemed reliable, and it is accurate to the best of the Author's knowledge; however, the Author cannot guarantee its accuracy and validity and cannot be held liable for any errors or omissions. Changes are periodically made to this book. You must consult your doctor or get professional medical advice before using any of the suggested remedies, techniques, or information in this book.

Upon using the information contained in this book, you agree to hold harmless the Author from and against any damages, costs, and expenses, including any legal fees potentially resulting from the application of any of the information provided by this guide. This disclaimer applies to any

2

damages or injury caused by the use and application, whether directly or indirectly, of any advice or information presented, whether for breach of contract, tort, negligence, personal injury, criminal intent, or under any other cause of action.

You agree to accept all risks of using the information presented inside this book. You need to consult a professional medical practitioner in order to ensure you are both able and healthy enough to participate in this program.

Table of Contents

Dinner Recipes 161

The 14-day DASH Diet Meal Plan:

Healthy Low-Sodium Recipes for Lower Blood Pressure and Weight Loss

By

Stephanie N. Collins

Introduction

In our world today, over a billion people are battling a prevalent, yet deadly disease condition that, unfortunately, is still on the rise. This disease is High Blood Pressure, also known as Hypertension.

One's choice of diet can cause or inhibit the growth of hypertension in the body. This goes to show there are diets that can help us manage and even prevent this disease.

Research has shown that individuals who have embraced plant-based diets, like vegetarians and vegans, usually have slim chances of suffering from High Blood Pressure.

Following up on this research, one type of diet, called the DASH diet, was initiated to help fight this disease, which is a significant contributor to kidney failure, heart failure, and stroke cases.

If you're hypertensive or you know someone who is, this book is for you, as it promises to show you all you need to know about Hypertension health.

Since staying informed is a primary duty, everybody should be intentional about it, particularly when it regards our health.

This book will not just give you all the background knowledge you need on Hypertension and how to deal with the disease; it will also show you the positive effects of a DASH diet.

Here are some things we'll be showing you in this book:

- What foods to eat and not to eat to maintain stable blood pressure.
- How to bring down high blood pressure levels.
- How to lose weight using a DASH diet.
- Why many people advocate this diet.
- How to cook with little amounts of sodium and still have tasty dishes.
- And a whole lot more.

Chapter 1: What You Need to Know About the DASH Diet

What is the DASH Diet?

DASH simply means Dietary Approaches to Stop Hypertension. This diet system was established by the United States National Institutes of Health.

The DASH diet is a lifelong method for maintaining a healthy diet.

Here are some proposed foods within the DASH diet:

- Fruits and vegetables
- Vegetable oils
- Whole grains
- Beans and nuts
- Poultry
- Fat-free and low-fat dairy foods

This diet places limitations on certain foods: foods with high levels of saturated fats, like full-fat dairy products and processed meats. Sweets and sweetened beverages are also on restriction, as well as tropical oils, like the palm and coconut oils. The DASH diet also advocates 2300 mg of sodium as the maximum daily intake for salt.

The DASH diet system has been proven by research to go a long way in the treatment and prevention of High Blood Pressure. Test results have also shown that further reducing the maximum daily salt intake to 1500 mg (lower sodium DASH diet) will further speed up the process of lowering high blood pressure in patients. This is a plus to what the regular DASH diet seeks to achieve.

Also, the DASH diet has been mentioned to help reduce cardio-metabolic risk measurements, specifically waist circumference, cholesterol levels, and weight. A DASH diet is generally regarded as a balanced diet system that ensures a healthy life when maintained.

Health Benefits of the DASH diet

Here are some significant health benefits of the DASH diet:

Reduced Blood Pressure levels

When the amount of sodium in the blood is more than it should be, it alters the sodium-potassium balance, which helps push out water from the bloodstream to the bladder, minimizing the kidney's ability to filter. This increased pressure is caused by the excess water in the blood, which in turn leads to an excess straining of the blood vessels that connect to the kidney, resulting in High Blood Pressure.

Since the DASH diet seeks to minimize the sodium intake levels in one's food, hypertension is thereby brought down in effect.

Prevent Osteoporosis

Living happily and maintaining a healthy life requires having healthy bones. Calcium, an essential component for strong bones among other mineral components, is lost through urine when there is excess sodium in the body. The DASH diet helps the body to regulate calcium loss, fostering stronger and healthier bones.

Prevent Cardiovascular Disease

Excess sodium in the body can cause significant harm to the heart and all the connecting arteries. At the early stages of hypertension, one observes a slight drop in the volume of blood reaching the heart, causing a sharp pain on the chest during activity.

This drop in the heart's blood flow results in an abnormality in its functions, owing to the short supply of oxygen and all the required nutrients in the blood. However, when blood pressure is brought down, it reduces the risk of such occurrences to the barest minimum. Hence, staying on a DASH diet ensures regulated blood pressure, which minimizes the chances of cardiovascular conditions.

Lowered Gout Risk

One other colossal profit of the DASH diet is its ability to bring down uric acid levels of hyperuricemia patients.

Such a balanced diet will naturally lower the occurrence of metabolic disorders, like a cerebrovascular disease, cardiovascular disease, and diabetes. This will result in a reduction in fat intake and an increase in the substitution of complex carbohydrates for simple sugars, leading to a lowering of both the total and the LDL cholesterols inside the blood, while lowering blood pressure.

Promotes Weight Loss

Although the DASH diet was basically created to help hypertensive patients, it was also discovered to aid weight loss.

Since the diet ensures minimized intake of added sugars and other processed foods, it is only natural that weight loss is achieved alongside enhanced metabolism.

Following all the recommendations of a DASH diet will result in reduced body fat, cardiovascular fitness, enhanced metabolism, increased strength, and loss of weight even without calorie counting.

Chapter 2: What to Eat and avoid on the DASH Diet

What to Eat

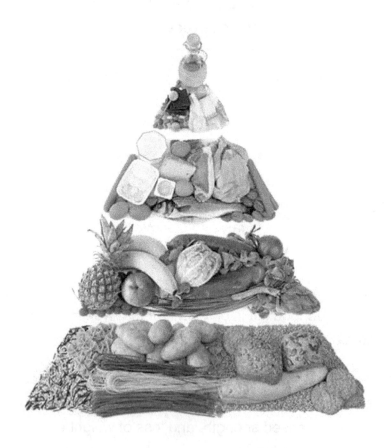

The DASH diet includes many veggies and fruits, whole grains, low-fat dairy, fish and poultry products, few legumes, red meat, sweets and a small number of fats in your day-to-day diet.

On this note, an individual eating the DASH diet requires typically 2000 kilocalories.

Recommended daily serving:

Whole Grains

Six to eight servings of whole grains, including bread, rice, and pasta.

What does one serving look like:

- 1 slice of whole -grain bread
- ½ cup cooked rice or pasta
- 1 oz. of dry cereal

Vegetables

Four to five servings of vegetables rich in fiber and vitamins.

What does one serving look like:

- ½ cup raw or cooked vegetable such as carrots, sweet potatoes, broccoli, tomatoes, mushrooms etc.
- 1 cup of raw leafy green veggies

Fruits

Four to five servings of fruits rich in magnesium, vitamins, fiber, potassium, and other minerals.

What does one serving look like:

- ½ cup of frozen, fresh or canned fruit (or berries)
- ¼ dried fruit
- 1 fresh medium fruit

Low-Fat Dairy Food

Dairy products are major sources of Vitamin D, protein, and calcium. You need 2-3 servings of low-fat dairy daily.

What does one serving look like:

- 1 cup (8 oz.) of skimmed milk or low-fat milk
- 1 cup of yogurt
- 1½ oz. of cheese

Lean Meat, Poultry, and Fish

As we all know, meat is an excellent source of vitamin B, proteins, zinc, and other valuable nutrients that are needed in the human body. Nevertheless, the DASH diet does not totally support the consumption of meat but recommends vegetables and fruits instead. Recommended day-to-day serving is 6 or less.

What does one serving look like:

- 1-2 oz. of cooked lean meat, skinless poultry or fish
- 1 egg

Nuts and Seeds

The DASH diet permits four to five (small servings) of seeds and nuts each week. What does one serving look like:

- ½ cup of cooked legumes
- 2 tablespoons of nut butter
- ⅓ cup of nuts
- 2 tablespoons of seeds

What to avoid

Sweets and added sugars

The consumption of sweets and added sugar should be minimally consumed while on the DASH diet. Try to limit the rate at which you take table sugar, soda, and candy to four or fewer times a week. Also, the DASH diet prohibits the use of unrefined sugars and all other sources of sugar, such as maple syrup, honey, and agave nectar.

Examples of a serving include:

- 1 tablespoon sugar

- 1 tablespoon jelly or jam

- 1 cup lemonade

Alcohol

Consumption of too much alcohol can damage the brain, heart, and liver and elevate blood pressure. Therefore, ensure to drink responsibly if you must drink at all.

Men are encouraged to cut down on their alcohol intake to two beverages per day and women one per day.

Chapter 3: Simple Steps to Improve Weight Loss and Blood Pressure

Steps to Regulating Blood Pressure and Weight Loss

Lifestyle plays an essential role in living a healthy and fit life, especially when you have been diagnosed with hypertension. If you have control over your high blood pressure via a healthy diet, there will be no need to take any type of medication as this could be a problem to most people.

Below are easy steps to start a healthier lifestyle to help reduce your high blood pressure through weight loss.

Step #1 – Watch Your Waistline

If you love watching your waistline, then you know when you're gaining some extra weight even without using a scale. As you add more weight, your blood pressure increases as well. Being overweight slows down your breathing rate while you're asleep, resulting in an imbalance to the blood pressure process.

Thus, to manage your blood pressure, one is advised to maintain a healthy waistline. Losing a little weight when you have gained too much or are obese can help in reducing your blood pressure by close to a millimeter of mercury with every pound of weight you cut down.

There are many health benefits when it comes to watching your waistline as having too much weight can create many health dangers. For men, having a waist that measures more than 102 centimeters or 40 inches can pose a risk. For women, having a waistline that is above 89 centimeters or 35 inches is a risk. However, note that these may differ among ethnic groups. Thus, you are advised to ask your health practitioner about this.

Step #2 – Have a Regular Exercise Regimen

Exercise is good for the body and has many benefits. Taking part in a regular physical activity, such as biking, brisk walking, or running, every morning before the day's task goes a long way in regulating your body's blood pressure.

Regular workouts help the heart perform optimally, improve your cognitive abilities, and enable the body to stay confident and strong to scale through the hurdles of life. Incorporate exercise activities in your daily or at least weekly schedule to help your body stay fit and regulate the body's blood pressure.

Step# 3 – Lower Your Salt Intake

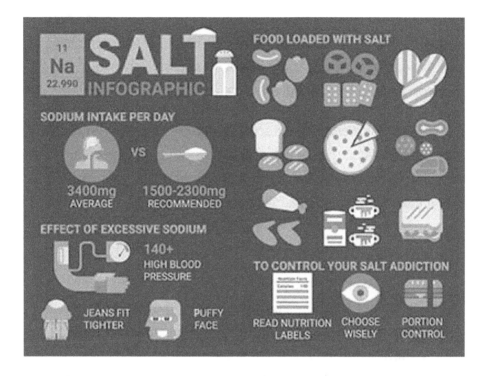

Reducing your salt intake level to the minimal can lower your blood pressure by close to 5-6 mm Hg if you are diagnosed with hypertension. Lowering your sodium intake can also benefit your heart health.

According to research, you should cut down your sodium intake to about 2300 mg daily or even less. Nevertheless, for those who are fully grown, consuming lower sodium of about 1500 mg each day or less is the best.

Before commencing the DASH diet, talk to your physician to get their opinion. It is of great significance that the diet works best for you based on your present health status. Although

DASH is the safest diet among all the popular diets we have today, your doctor's opinion is still needed. After all, there are two different options of the DASH diet to choose from. You may prefer the option that needs 1500 mg of sodium intake in a day or the 2300 mg daily intake of sodium, and your physician knows exactly what fits your body.

If you do not monitor your sodium intake, you may be advised by your physician to begin at a higher level. Nevertheless, as soon as you are aware of the salt contained in your meal, you can then start to reduce the level of consumption. According to your salt intake, consider the following tips:

Consuming Less Salt

A teaspoon of salt houses about 2300 mg of sodium, which isn't good for a hypertension patient. To stay away from all these health dangers, cut down the amount of salt you consume daily and stick to the DASH diet. Preferably, herbs and spices can take the place of salt in your meals.

If you are used to consuming salt, then gradually reduce the amount of salt you add to your meal, and with time, you will get used to meals without salt.

Reading Labels

Labels have been attached to most food products for the buyer's benefit. If you love buying packed processed food, then you are more likely to consume a high amount of sodium. When buying packed instant food, carefully study the labels to ensure you are aware of the amount of sodium you will be taking in to avoid future inconveniences. You will find the amount of sodium at the bottom of all labels.

Step #4- Eat Recommended DASH Diet Foods

As soon as you can cut down your sodium consumption, it is time to stick to the DASH diet completely. The DASH diet method is discussed throughout this book, though to make it more transparent, consume foods with the following contents:

- Rich in whole grains, vegetables, and fruits.

- Limited fat and cholesterol

- Low-fat dairy products

Follow Nutritional Guide

As soon as you can cut down your sodium intake to the levels recommended by doctors while eating the DASH diet, then you can control your nutrient intake. It has been claimed by the National Institute of Researchers that those who stick to the DASH diet met their nutritional goals and succeeded in losing weight and improving their blood pressure in the process.

- Cholesterol (150 mg)
- Protein (18%)
- Carbohydrates (55%)
- Total Fat (27%)
- Sodium (2300 mg)

- Saturated Fat (6%)
- Potassium (4700 mg)
- Calcium (1250 mg)
- Magnesium (500 mg)
- Fiber (30 g)
- Calcium (1250 mg)

Daily Caloric Requirements

DASH Diet Daily Calorie Requirement for Men			
Age (in Years)	Sedentary Men (Calories /day)	Moderately Active Men Calories /day)	Active Men (Calories /day)
19-30	2400	2600-2800	3000
31-50	2200	2400-2600	2800-3000
50 and above	2000	2200-2400	2400-2800

DASH Diet Daily Calorie Requirement for Women			
Age (in Years)	Sedentary Women (Calories /day)	Moderately Active Women Calories /day)	Active Women (Calories /day)
19-30	2000	2000-2200	2400
31-50	1800	2000	2200
50 and above	1600	1800	2000-2200

DASH Diet Food Group Servings/Day for Women and Men							
Food Group	1200 Cal	1400 Cal	1600 Cal	1800 Cal	2000 Cal	2600 Cal	3100 Cal
Veggies	3-4	3-4	3-4	4-5	4-5	5-6	6
Fruits	3-4	4	4	4-5	4-5	5-6	6
Grains	4-5	5-6	6	6	6-8	10-11	12-13
Meet, Poultry, and Fish	3 or less	3-4 or less	3-4 or less	6 or less	6 or less	6 or less	6-9
Low-Fat and Fat-Free Dairy	2-3	2-3	2-3	2-3	2-3	3	3-4
Nuts, Legumes, and Seeds	3 per week	3 per week	3-4 per week	4 per week	4-5 per week	1	1
Healthy Fats and Oils	1	1	2	2-3	2-3	3	4
Maximum Sodium	2300 mg per day	2300 mg per day	2300 mg per day	2300 mg per day	2300 mg per day	2300 mg per day	2300 mg per day
Sweets and Sugar	3 or less per week	3 or less per week	3 or less per week	3 or less per week	3 or less per week	3 or less per week	3 or less per week

Step #5 - Limit Alcohol and Quit Smoking

Limiting alcohol consumption can potentially reduce your hypertension by 4 mm Hg; this means that drinking alcohol regularly can distort a person's normal blood pressure level. For women, just a cup of liquor can be consumed per day, while for men, a maximum of two is the limit per day.

Taking more than the average amount of alcohol can increase your blood pressure level, and this is bad for those with hypertension, as it affects the effectiveness of all blood pressure drugs.

Just like alcohol, the same applies to smoking. Just one cigarette can cause immeasurable harm to your blood pressure. Here is the good news; quitting smoking can help return your blood pressure to the normal level. When you stop

31

smoking, you reduce your risk of lung and heart disease and increase your chances of staying healthier and stronger than every other smoker.

Step #6 - Cut Back on Caffeine

The impact of caffeine on blood pressure is still debatable. For people who rarely consume caffeine, it causes the blood pressure to rise to 10 mm Hg, but for those who regularly drink coffee, it can either have little or no effect at all.

Although caffeine's long-term effect on blood pressure is still unclear, there is the possibility that blood pressure may increase by 5-10 mg Hg if you are sensitive to the blood-raising effects of caffeine.

Step #7 - Manage Stress

Chronic stress can have a significant impact on high blood pressure. Even occasional stress may likewise raise your blood pressure level if your response is eating unhealthy food, smoking, or drinking alcohol more than the moderate level.

Consider an effective stress management strategy that can help you combat stress. Make sure to observe a balanced and healthy lifestyle.

Chapter 4: DASH Diet Tips

There are a certain number of servings of different food groups required by the DASH diet per day. There may be a variation when it comes to the number of meals based on your needed day-to-day calorie consumption, which can help you make changes.

For example, you cut down your day-to-day sodium consumption to just a teaspoon full of salt or 2400 mg. When your body gets used to the diet, you can reduce your sodium intake to as low as half a teaspoon or 1500 mg. This amount should comprise every sodium content of your diet and the extra ingredients you place on the table when eating.

Below are a few easy tips to increase the many benefits of the DASH diet.

- Include a serving of fruits and vegetables at every meal, even when eating snacks.
- Utilize low-fat or fat-free condiments.
- Always inspect the label of any food product you buy to see that dried and canned fruits are low in sodium and do not include added sugar content.
- Make use of only half the regular servings of salad dressing, margarine, or butter.
- Cut down your meat consumption to six ounces daily or add chicken to your meal twice or three times each week.
- When it is meal time, include dry beans in your diet.

- While you love eating snacks and all other kinds of junk foods, chips, or sweets, try consuming pretzels, unsalted nuts, or raisins. Also, consume plain popcorn that contains zero butter.
- Invest more in organic fruits and vegetables from the farmer's market.
- Invest in fish or meat from local fish sellers or slaughterhouses.
- Throw away all processed food substances in your kitchen.
- Quit smoking.
- Minimize your intake of caffeine and alcohol.
- Engage in healthy exercises.
- Try as much as you can to avoid junk foods and fast food.

Simple Ways to Add Flavor without Salt

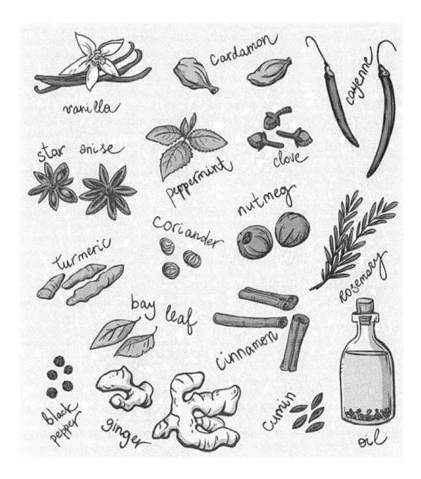

At this level, you should know that excess consumption of sodium can pose as a starting point for stroke and increase your blood pressure. If you find it hard to stay away from sodium completely, there are other methods and ways to cut down your consumption of sodium and still have a delicious meal at the same time. Below are a few ingredients you can add to your meal to make it taste good even without including salt.

Ginger

With ginger's unique flavor that's both spicy and sweet, you can blend it with any protein, including chicken, pork, fish, and other forms of meat, to double the dish's flavor and health benefits.

The anti-inflammatory compound in ginger, called gingerols, can bring relief and mobility to those suffering from arthritis, while providing protection from damage brought about by free radicals.

With ginger's super-great flavor, which is sweet and spicy, you can easily combine it with protein-filled meals, such as fish, chicken, pork, and all other sources of meat, to add to your health benefits and the flavor of your dish.

Parsley

Parsley is a leafy ingredient. You can find parsley all year round. Adding this abundant ingredient to your stews and soups will introduce an intricate and fresh taste to all delicious meals. This leafy ingredient is available throughout all seasons. Try not to mince your parsley, as this will reduce the flavor when chewing it.

Parsley is Vitamin K enriched, and it helps with blood clotting and keeping your bones healthy.

Cilantro

Most people enjoy tasting cilantro in their dishes, while others hate adding this flavor to their meals. Are you a fan of cilantro? Add it to rice and stir-fried dishes.

Rosemary

The tasty flavor rosemary adds to your sauce will make you eat more if you're a lover of pasta.

If you prefer sautéing your meals, you'll love the yummy taste of whole sprigs of rosemary and garlic spiced oil while making your favorite dish. Believe me, even Grandma will be tempted to have a bite after inhaling its irresistible aroma as you serve the meal.

Aside from the memorable experience rosemary offers, this secret ingredient serves as a natural treat for heartburn and a quick digestion aid.

Combination of Herbs

Combining one single herb, such as oregano or rosemary, with twice as much parsley (for instance) is a way of spicing up your egg dishes and roasted potatoes.

Experimenting with different types of flavors will help you get the right taste for some special meals. You can combine mild-flavored herbs, such as basil and chives, with strong-flavored ones, such as rosemary, to create a flavor-enhanced dish even with less salt.

Chapter 5: 14-Day DASH Diet Menu to Lose Weight and Lower Blood Pressure

	BREAKFAST	LUNCH	DINNER
Day 1	Peanut Butter Oats in a Jar	Salmon & Asparagus Stew with Farro	Dash Steak Salad with Roasted Corn Dressing
Day 2	Healthy Blueberry & Banana Muffins	Nutritious Vegetable Soup	Spiced Beef Kebobs
Day 3	Heart-Friendly Sweet Potato-Oats Waffles	Citrusy Grilled Tilapia & Pineapple Salsa	Simple Dash Strawberry Salad
Day 4	Simple Tofu Breakfast Scramble	Greek Quinoa Bowl	Wholesome Vegetable Pizza
Day 5	Spinach-Mushroom Omelet	Chicken-Orange Heart-Friendly Tortilla	Tomato & Corn Cheese Tortellini
Day 6	Chocolate-Berry Banana Smoothie	Dash Diet Pork Chops with Mustard	Summer Salad with Grilled Shrimp
Day 7	Yummy Dash Egg Salad	Herby Baked Salmon	Baked Broccoli & Cauliflower with Piquant Yogurt Sauce
Day 8	Wholesome Portobello Mushroom Florentine	Quick & Easy Balsamic Chicken with Veggies	Orange, Beet & Ricotta Salad
Day 9	Energizing Quinoa Bars	Baked Halibut and Tomato Salsa	Dash Chicken Chili
Day 10	Apples & Steel-Cut Oats	Nutty Spinach & Blue Cheese Salad	Healthy Ziti & Meatballs
Day 11	Simple Vegan Buckwheat Crepes	Cheesy Chicken & Spinach Tortilla	Quick & Easy Avocado Salad
Day 12	Banana Cinnamon & Peanut Butter	Autumn-Flavored Spinach Salad	Apricot-Glazed Balsamic Turkey
Day 13	Healthy Breakfast Toast	Teriyaki Salmon & Broccoli	Ultimate Dash Burger
Day 14	Cauliflower Breakfast Patties	Healthy Pomegranate & Ricotta	Lemony and Peppery Tuna Steak

Chapter 6: DASH Recipes

Breakfast

Peanut Butter Oats in the Jar

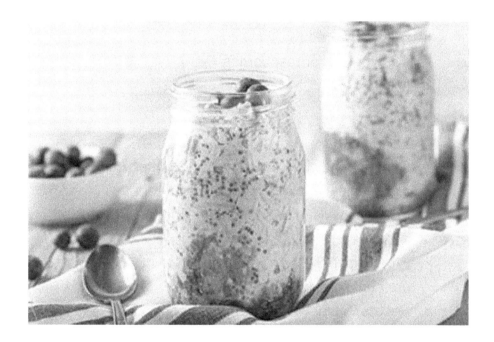

Preparation Time: 6 hours and 5 minutes

Yield: 1 serving

Ingredients

For the oats:

- ½ cup gluten-free rolled oats

- ½ cup unsweetened, plain almond milk
- 4 tablespoons natural salted peanut butter
- 1 tablespoon maple syrup (or stevia, organic brown sugar)
- ¾ tablespoon chia seeds

For the toppings (optional):

- Banana, sliced
- Strawberries or raspberries
- Chia seeds

Directions

1. Combine the almond milk, peanut butter, chia seeds, and maple syrup in a Mason jar. Stir but don't over-mix to leave swirls of peanut butter. Add the oats and stir again.
2. Press down the oats with a spoon to make sure they are soaked in the milk mixture.
3. Secure the jar with a lid and refrigerate for at least 6 hours.
4. To serve, garnish with toppings of choice.

Note: Nutritional info does not include toppings.

Nutrition Facts

Per serving (1 Mason jar) | Calories: 454 | Carbohydrates: 50.9g | Fat: 3.9g | Saturated Fat: 2g | Fiber: 12g | Protein: 14.6g | Sodium: 162mg | Sugar: 14.9g

Heart-Friendly Sweet Potato-Oats Waffles

Preparation Time: 5 minutes

Cooking Time: 10 minutes

Yield: 6 medium waffles

Ingredients

For the waffles:

- 1 cup rolled oats
- ½ cup sweet potato, cooked and skin removed
- 1 whole egg
- 1 egg white
- 1 cup almond milk
- 1 tablespoon honey
- 1 tablespoon olive oil
- ¼ teaspoon baking powder
- ¼ teaspoon salt

To serve:

- Banana, sliced
- Maple syrup

Directions

1. Preheat the waffle iron.

2. Meanwhile, add all the ingredients to a blender and process until pureed. Let the mixture stand for 10 minutes.
3. Coat the waffle iron with a nonstick cooking spray.
4. Pour $\frac{1}{3}$ cup of the batter in each mold. Cook about 3-4 minutes per batch or 30 seconds longer after the light indicator turns green. Usually, waffles are done after the steam stops coming out of the waffle iron.
5. Serve with banana slices and maple syrup on top.

Nutrition Facts

Per serving (2 waffles) | Calories: 287 | Carbohydrates: 54g | Fat: 8.39g | Saturated Fat: 1.6g | Fiber: 7.2g | Protein: 12.42g | Sodium: 285mg | Sugar: 22g

Simple Tofu Breakfast Scramble

Preparation Time: 10 minutes

Cooking Time: 20 minutes

Yield: 2 servings

Ingredients

For the scramble:

- 2 cups kale, roughly chopped
- 8 oz. extra-firm tofu
- ¼ red onion, thinly sliced
- ½ red pepper, thinly sliced
- 1-2 tablespoons olive oil

For the sauce:

- ½ teaspoon garlic powder
- ¼ teaspoon chili powder
- ½ teaspoon cumin powder
- ¼ teaspoon turmeric (optional)
- ½ teaspoon sea salt
- Water, for thinning

To serve (optional):

- Salsa

- Cilantro
- Fruits

Directions

1. Pat the tofu dry using a paper towel and roll in a clean kitchen towel. Put something heavy (e.g., cast iron skillet) on top and leave it for about 15 minutes.
2. Meanwhile, prepare the sauce by combining the spices and salt in a small bowl. Add enough water for a pourable consistency.
3. Heat oil in a large skillet placed over medium heat. Sauté the onions and red pepper then season with salt. Continue to cook about 5 minutes or until the veggies are tender.
4. Add the kale, a bit more salt, and pepper then cover with a lid. Continue to cook for another 2 minutes.
5. Place the tofu on a plate and crumble into bite-sized pieces with a fork.
6. Uncover the skillet and move the veggies on one side of the pan with a spatula. Add the tofu and sauté 2 minutes. Add the sauce, pouring more of it over the tofu and just a bit over the veggies. Stir and cook another 5-7 minutes or until the tofu is slightly browned.
7. Serve with salsa, cilantro, and/or fruits if desired. You also can store it in a freezer for up to a month.

Note: Nutritional info does not include side dish.

Nutrition Facts

Per serving (about 170g) | Calories: 252 | Carbohydrates: 12.7g | Fat: 19g | Saturated Fat: 3g | Fiber: 3g | Protein: 12g | Sodium: 516mg | Sugar: 2.5g

Chocolate-Berry Banana Smoothie

Preparation Time: 5 minutes

Yield: 1 serving

Ingredients

- ½ cup fresh (or frozen) berries of choice
- ⅛ cup unsweetened cocoa powder
- 1 medium banana, peeled
- 1 cup vanilla soy milk
- 1 teaspoon chia seeds
- 1 DASH ground cinnamon
- 1 DASH ground nutmeg

Directions

1. Place all the ingredients in a blender or food processor then pulse until smooth. Serve immediately.

Nutrition Facts

Per serving (12 ounces) | Calories: 252 | Carbohydrates: 33g | Fat: 12g | Saturated Fat: 2g | Fiber: 8g | Protein: 11g | Sodium: 102mg | Sugar: 8g

Healthy Blueberry & Banana Muffins

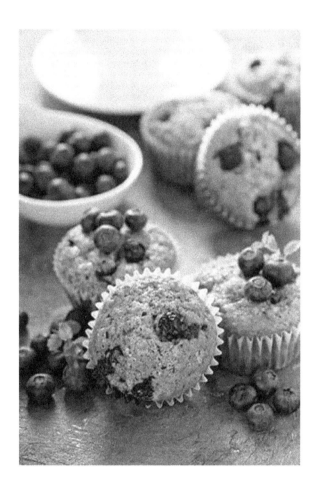

Preparation Time: 20 minutes

Cooking Time: 25 minutes

Yield: 12 large muffins

Ingredients

- 1¼ cups frozen (or fresh) blueberries

- ¾ cup (about 2 medium) ripe banana, mashed
- ¾ cup + 2 tablespoons unsweetened almond milk
- 2 cups white-spelt flour
- ¼ cup pure maple syrup
- ¼ cup coconut oil, melted
- 4 -6 tablespoons coconut sugar (or natural cane sugar)
- 1 teaspoon apple cider vinegar
- 1 teaspoon pure vanilla extract
- 2 teaspoons baking powder
- 1½ teaspoons cinnamon
- ½ teaspoon fine-grain sea salt
- ½ teaspoon baking soda
- ½ cup walnut halves, chopped (optional)

Directions

1. Preheat oven to 350°F and lightly coat a muffin tin with a nonstick cooking spray.
2. In a medium bowl, incorporate the mashed bananas, milk, maple syrup, apple cider vinegar, vanilla, and coconut oil.
3. In a large bowl, add the flour, sugar, baking soda, baking powder, cinnamon, and salt.
4. Add the wet mixture into the dry mixture. Stir enough to combine. Do not overmix, since the spelt flour is fragile.
5. Gently fold in the nuts (if using) and then the blueberries, making sure not to overmix since this will produce hard muffins.

6. Pour about ¼ cup of batter into each muffin tin slot, filling about ¾ full. Press a few blueberries on top if desired.
7. Bake at 350°F for about 23-27 minutes. Perform a toothpick test to check if it's done.
8. Let cool for about 5-8 minutes. Transfer the muffins to a cooling rack and cool for an additional 15 minutes.

Nutrition Facts

Per serving (1 muffin) | Calories: 180 | Carbohydrates: 31g |Fat: 5g | Saturated Fat: 4g | Fiber: 2g | Protein: 4g | Sodium: 160mg | Sugar: 12g

Yummy DASH Egg Salad

Preparation Time: 5 minutes

Cooking Time: 10 minutes

Yield: 1 serving

Ingredients

- 1½ cups arugula (or lettuce, spinach), torn
- 2 hard-boiled eggs, diced
- ½ sweet bell pepper (any color), cubed
- ½ medium tomato, cubed
- ½ baby cucumber, cubed
- 1 tablespoon (about ⅛) avocado, diced
- 1 oz. non-fat mozzarella cheese, cubed
- 1 teaspoon thyme, crushed
- 1 teaspoon olive oil

Directions

1. In a large bowl, add the arugula, cucumber, bell pepper, tomato, eggs, avocado, mozzarella, and thyme. Drizzle with olive oil and toss.

Nutrition Facts

Per serving (about 578g) | Calories: 568 | Carbohydrates: 15.9 | Fat: 35.31g | Saturated Fat: 9.8g | Fiber: 3.8g | Protein: 45.7g | Sodium: 556mg | Sugar: 6.88g

Wholesome Portobello Mushroom Florentine

Preparation Time: 3 minutes

Cooking Time: 22 minutes

Yield: 2 servings

Ingredients

- 2 large Portobello mushrooms
- 1 cup fresh baby spinach
- ¼ cup goat or feta cheese, crumbled
- 1 small onion, chopped
- 2 large eggs, beaten
- Fresh basil, minced
- ½ teaspoon olive oil
- ⅛ teaspoon pepper
- ⅛ teaspoon garlic salt
- Pinch of salt

Directions

1. Preheat oven to 425°F. Clean the mushrooms with a clean, damp cloth and remove their stems.
2. Spritz the mushrooms with cooking spray and arrange them in a 15x10-inch pan with the stem-side up. Season with garlic salt and pepper.
3. Bake the mushrooms uncovered for about 10 minutes or until tender.

4. Heat the oil in a nonstick skillet placed over medium-high heat. Cook the onion until tender. Add the spinach; stir and cook until wilted.
5. Season the beaten eggs with salt and add to the skillet. Cook until the eggs thicken, stirring until they're set.
6. Spoon the egg mixture into the mushrooms. To serve, sprinkle with cheese and basil.

Nutrition Facts

Per serving (1 stuffed mushroom) | Calories: 126 | Carbohydrates: 10g | Fat: 5g | Saturated Fat: 2g | Fiber: 3g | Protein: 11g | Sodium: 472mg | Sugar: 4g

Slow-Cooked Energizing Quinoa Bars

Preparation Time: 10 minutes

Cooking Time: 4 hours

Yield: 8 bars

Ingredients

- ⅓ cup quinoa uncooked
- ⅓ cup dried apples, roughly chopped
- ⅓ cup roasted almonds, roughly chopped
- 1 cup unsweetened vanilla almond milk
- 2 large eggs
- ½ cup raisins
- ½ teaspoon cinnamon
- 2 tablespoons chia seeds
- 2 tablespoons pure maple syrup
- 2 tablespoons almond butter (plus more for drizzling)
- Pinch of salt

Directions

1. Coat the 5-quart slow cooker with a nonstick cooking spray. Cut a piece of parchment to fit at the bottom of the crock. Spritz the parchment with cooking spray as well.
2. Combine the almond butter and maple syrup in a large microwave-safe bowl. Microwave it for about 30

seconds until the butter is creamy. Once done, stir the mixture.

3. Add the almond milk, salt, and cinnamon to the butter mixture. Stir until well-combined.
4. Stir in the eggs then all the remaining ingredients. Make sure everything is incorporated completely.
5. Pour the mixture into the cooker and set on "low". Cook about $3\frac{1}{2}$ to 4 hours or until the top of the quinoa mixture is set. Turn off the cooker and take the lid off, letting the quinoa cool inside completely.
6. Run the knife around the quinoa edges and remove from the cooker.
7. Divide and cut into 8 pieces. Drizzle with almond butter and serve.

Nutrition Facts

Per serving (71g) | Calories: 174 | Carbohydrates: 20.1g | Fat: 8.4g | Saturated Fat: 1.1g | Fiber: 4.3g | Protein: 6.1g | Sodium: 39mg | Sugar: 9.1g

Spinach-Mushroom Omelet

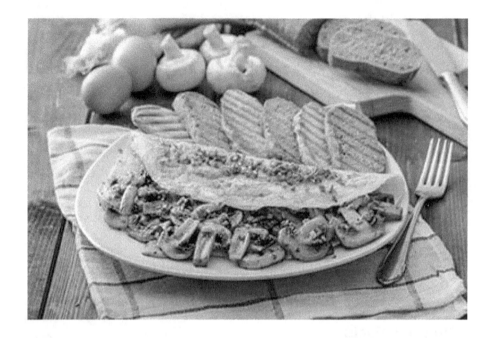

Preparation Time: 3 minutes

Cooking Time: 15 minutes

Yield: 1 serving

Ingredients

- 5 baby Bella mushrooms, sliced
- ¼ cup red onion, sliced
- 1½ cups fresh spinach
- 1 oz. goat cheese
- 1 whole egg
- 2 egg whites

- 1 tablespoon olive oil
- Green onions, diced (optional, for garnish)

Directions

1. Put a medium skillet over medium-high flame and add the oil. Once the oil is hot, add the onions and sauté about 2-3 minutes or until translucent.
2. Add the mushrooms. Cook for about 4-5 minutes or until they are slightly browned.
3. Add the spinach and cook until it's wilted. Season with salt and pepper then set aside.
4. Place a small skillet over medium heat and coat with a nonstick cooking spray.
5. Add the whole egg and egg whites in a small bowl and whisk to combine.
6. Pour the egg mixture into the small skillet. Let it sit for about a minute before running a spatula around the edges of the omelet. Lift the skillet and tilt it down for a bit until the still-runny eggs slide to the edge of the pan. Once there, carefully swirl the skillet, letting the liquid part become cooked around the edges. Cook for another minute.
7. Carefully add the spinach-mushroom mixture and crumbled goat cheese to one side of the omelet. Cook for half a minute and fold the empty side of the omelet over the side with toppings.
8. Transfer the omelet to a serving plate. Garnish with green onions if desired.

Nutrition Facts

Per serving (1 omelet) | Calories: 412 | Carbohydrates: 18g |
Fat: 29g | Saturated Fat: 10g | Fiber: 4g | Protein: 25g |
Sodium: 332mg | Sugar: 8g

Apples & Steel-Cut Oats

Preparation Time: 10 minutes

Cooking Time: 10 hours

Yield: 8 servings

Ingredients

For the oats:

- 2 cups steel-cut oats
- 2 cups apples, chopped
- 1 cup low-fat milk
- 1 cup dried cranberries
- 3 cups water
- 2 teaspoons margarine
- 1 tablespoon cinnamon, ground
- 1 teaspoon pumpkin pie spice

For toppings (optional):

- ½ cup almonds, sliced
- ½ cup pecans

Directions

1. Coat the slow cooker crock with margarine.
2. Place all the ingredients (except for the nuts) into the slow cooker. Stir to combine.

3. Set the cooker to "warm" and cook for about 10 hours. Before serving, top with nuts if desired.

Nutrition Facts

Per serving (about 200g) | Calories: 264.5 | Carbohydrates: 47.8g | Fat: 7.1g | Saturated Fat: 1.1g | Fiber: 6.9g | Protein: 8.4g | Sodium: 28.7mg | Sugar: 11.8g

Simple Vegan Buckwheat Crepes with Strawberry Compote

Preparation Time: 10 minutes

Cooking Time: 15 minutes

Yield: 12 crepes

Ingredients

For the crepes:

- 1 cup raw buckwheat flour
- ¾ tablespoon flaxseed meal
- 1¾ cups light-canned coconut milk
- 1 pinch sea salt
- 1 tablespoon avocado oil
- ⅛ teaspoon ground cinnamon (optional)

For the compote:

- 3 cups fresh (or frozen) strawberries
- 3 tablespoons orange juice

Directions

1. For the crepes, process the buckwheat flour, coconut milk, cinnamon, flaxseed, avocado oil, and salt in a blender. Once done, the batter should be pourable but

not watery. If the batter is too thick, add more milk. If too thin, add a little more buckwheat flour.

2. Place a nonstick skillet over medium heat. Once hot, brush the surface with a thin layer of oil. Heat the oil then add $\frac{1}{4}$ cup batter. Cook until the top becomes bubbly and the edges are dry. Flip the crepe with a spatula and cook another 2-3 minutes. Repeat until all crepes are done.

3. For the compote, put the strawberries and juice in a small saucepan over medium heat. Once bubbling, reduce the heat to medium-low.

4. Mash the strawberries with a wooden spoon and continue to cook about 10-12 minutes. Mash the fruit occasionally as you cook.

5. Turn off the heat and let the compote cool for a bit. Transfer to a clean jar and let the compote cool completely.

6. Serve the crepes with the compote.

Nutrition Facts

Per serving (1 crepe with 2 tablespoons compote) | Calories: 86 | Carbohydrates: 15.55g | Fat: 2.34g | Saturated Fat: 0.23g | Fiber: 2.1g | Protein: 2g | Sodium: 30mg | Sugar: 6.9g

Healthy Breakfast Toast

Preparation Time: 8-10 minutes

Cooking Time: 8-10 minutes

Yield: 1 serving

Ingredients

- 1 slice whole-grain bread, toasted
- 2 cups baby spinach
- ½ small avocado, mashed
- 1 large egg
- 1 tablespoon salsa
- 1 teaspoon extra-virgin olive oil, divided
- 1 clove garlic, minced
- Pinch of ground pepper

Directions

1. Spread the mashed avocado on the toast. Season with ground pepper.
2. Place a small nonstick skillet over medium heat and add ½ teaspoon olive oil. Sauté the garlic and spinach for about one minute, stirring it continuously until wilted. Transfer the spinach on top of the toast.
3. Add the remaining half teaspoon of oil to the skillet. Cook the egg over medium-low heat for about 5-7 minutes or until the yolk is set but still runny. Once done, transfer it onto the top of spinach.

4. Last, top the egg with salsa.

Nutrition Facts

Per serving (1 toast) | Calories: 364 | Carbohydrates: 24g |
Fat: 26g | Saturated Fat: 5g | Fiber: 10g | Protein: 14g |
Sodium: 330mg | Sugar: 3g

Banana Cinnamon & Peanut Butter Toast

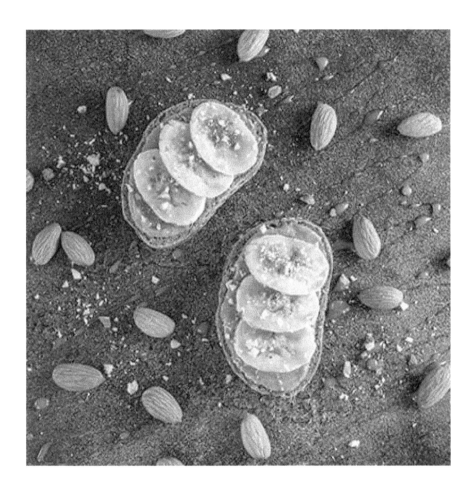

Preparation Time: 5 minutes

Yield: 1 serving

Ingredients

- 1 slice whole-wheat bread, toasted
- 1 small banana, sliced
- 1 tablespoon peanut butter

- Pinch of cinnamon

Directions

1. Put peanut butter on one side of the toast. Top with banana slices and sprinkle with cinnamon.

Nutrition Facts

Per serving (1 toast) | Calories: 266 | Carbohydrates: 38g | Fat: 9g | Saturated Fat: 2g | Fiber: 5g | Protein: 8g | Sodium: 181mg | Sugar: 14g

Cauliflower Breakfast Patties

Preparation Time: 5 minutes

Cooking Time: 35 minutes

Yield: 4 servings

Ingredients

- ½ medium head cauliflower
- 1 large egg
- ½ cup onion, finely chopped
- 1 cup fat-free cheddar, shredded
- 3 tablespoons cornstarch
- 1 tablespoon extra-virgin olive oil
- Freshly ground black pepper
- Pinch of salt

Directions

1. Shred the cauliflower using a box grater and place in a medium bowl. Add the cheese, egg, onion, cornstarch, salt, and pepper.
2. Put a large skillet over medium-high heat then add the oil.
3. When the oil is hot enough, add spoons of cauliflower mixture and shape into a patty. Fry until golden brown and crispy, about 5 minutes per side. Transfer to a plate and serve hot.

Nutrition Facts

Per serving (1 patty) | Calories: 129 | Carbohydrates: 10.85g |
Fat: 4.61g | Saturated Fat: 0.9g | Fiber: 1g | Protein: 11.52g |
Sodium: 326mg | Sugar: 1.27g

Lunch

DASH Diet Pork Chops with Mustard Sauce

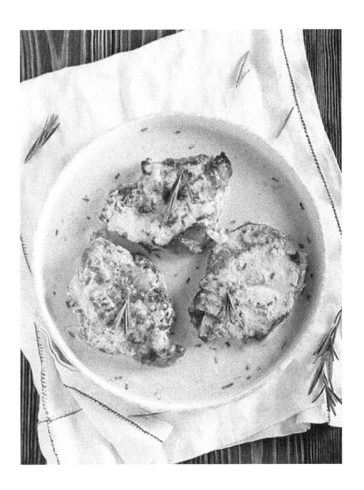

Preparation Time: 5 minutes

Cooking Time: 25 minutes

Yield: 4 servings

Ingredients

- 4 boneless pork chops
- ½ cup low-sodium chicken broth
- ½ cup low-fat milk
- 2 tablespoons onion, minced
- 1 tablespoon Dijon mustard
- 1 tablespoon unsalted butter
- 2 teaspoons rosemary
- 2 teaspoons cornstarch
- 2 tablespoons canola oil
- ¼ teaspoon black pepper
- Pinch of salt

Directions

1. Heat oil in a large skillet placed over medium heat. Rub the pork chops with salt and pepper then add to the skillet.
2. Cook each side of the pork chops about 3 minutes or until golden brown. Once done, the meat should be firm at the thickest part when pressed. Transfer to a plate and set aside.
3. Stir cornstarch into the broth then add milk and mustard. Stir well to combine and set aside.
4. In the same skillet, melt the butter over medium heat and sauté the onions until tender.
5. Stir the cornstarch-broth mixture again. Carefully pour into the skillet and bring it to a boil.

6. Transfer the pork chops together with its juices (if there are any) into the skillet and cook. Turn them occasionally until the sauce becomes thick.
7. Transfer the pork to plates and cut each chop using a knife. Spoon the sauce over the pork chops and garnish with rosemary before serving.

Nutrition Facts

Per serving (1 pork chop) | Calories: 353 | Carbohydrates: 3.66g | Fat: 17.15g | Saturated Fat: 5.02g | Fiber: 0.3g | Protein: 43.34g | Sodium: 256mg | Sugar: 1.82g

Greek Quinoa Bowl

Preparation Time: 7 minutes

Cooking Time: 23 minutes

Yield: 4 servings

Ingredients

- 1 cup quinoa, rinsed and well drained
- ¾ cup canned garbanzo beans or chickpeas, rinsed and drained
- ½ cup crumbled feta cheese
- ¼ cup Greek olives, finely chopped
- 1 medium zucchini, chopped
- 1 medium tomato, finely chopped
- 2 cups water
- 2 cloves garlic, minced
- 2 tablespoons fresh basil, minced
- 1 tablespoon olive oil
- ¼ teaspoon black pepper

Directions

1. Heat oil in a large saucepan placed over medium-high heat. Once hot, add the garlic and quinoa; cook about 2-3 minutes, stirring frequently. When the quinoa turns lightly brown, stir in the water and zucchini then bring the mixture to a boil.

2. Adjust the heat to medium, cover the saucepan with lid, and let simmer for 12-15 minutes or until the liquid is absorbed.
3. Add the rest of the ingredients and heat through. Transfer into bowls and serve hot.

Nutrition Facts

Per serving (1 cup) | Calories: 310 | Carbohydrates: 42g | Fat: 11g | Saturated Fat: 3g | Fiber: 6g | Protein: 11g | Sodium: 353mg | Sugar: 3g

Salmon & Asparagus Stew with Farro

Preparation Time: 10 minutes

Cooking Time: 40 minutes

Yield: 4 servings

Ingredients

- 1¼ lbs. wild Alaskan salmon fillet, skinned and cut into 1-inch cubes
- ¾ cup farro
- 1 bunch asparagus
- 2 cups leeks (white and light green parts only), halved and thinly sliced
- 2 cups low-sodium chicken broth
- 3 cups water
- 2 cloves garlic, minced
- 3 tablespoons white miso
- 3 tablespoons fresh basil, very thinly sliced
- 1 tablespoon extra-virgin olive oil
- ¼ teaspoon pepper

Directions

1. Trim the asparagus and cut into 1-inch pieces.
2. In a medium saucepan, combine the farro and water. Set the stove to high heat and bring the farro to a boil. Reduce the heat to medium-low and cover the

saucepan with a lid. Cook another 30 minutes or until tender and chewy. Drain.

3. About 15 minutes after starting to cook the farro, place a large saucepan over medium heat. Pour the oil. Once hot, sauté leeks for about 2 minutes, stirring often, until soft.

4. Add the garlic and asparagus. Stir continuously for another 2 minutes or until the asparagus turns bright green.

5. Add the miso and broth, adjust the heat to high, and bring it to a boil.

6. Adjust the heat to medium and add the salmon. Stir gently and let simmer for about 3 minutes.

7. Turn off the heat and stir in the basil and pepper.

8. Divide the farro among 4 bowls and scoop the salmon stew on top of the farro.

Nutrition Facts

Per serving (1½ cups stew and ½ cup farro) | Calories: 407 | Carbohydrates: 40g | Fat: 11g | Saturated Fat: 2g | Fiber: 5g | Protein: 37g | Sodium: 432mg | Sugar: 4g

Nutritious Vegetable Soup

Preparation Time: 10 minutes

Cooking Time: 35 minutes

Yield: 9 servings

Ingredients

- 1 lb. fresh green beans, cut into 1-inch pieces
- 1 cup carrots, chopped
- 1 cup onion, chopped
- 6 cups reduced-sodium chicken or vegetable broth
- ¼ cup fresh basil, minced
- 2 teaspoons butter
- 1 clove garlic, minced
- 3 cups fresh tomatoes, diced
- ½ teaspoon salt
- ¼ teaspoon black pepper

Directions

1. Place a large saucepan over medium heat. Add the butter and sauté the carrots and onions for about 5 minutes.
2. Add the broth, garlic, and beans then stir. Bring it to a boil, reduce the heat, and let it simmer with the lid on for about 20 minutes or until the vegetables are tender.

3. Add the basil, tomatoes, salt, and pepper. Put the lid on again and simmer another 5 minutes.

Nutrition Facts

Per serving (1 cup) | Calories: 58 | Carbohydrates: 10g | Fat: 1g | Saturated Fat: 1g | Fiber: 3g | Protein: 4g | Sodium: 535mg | Sugar: 5g

Herby Baked Salmon

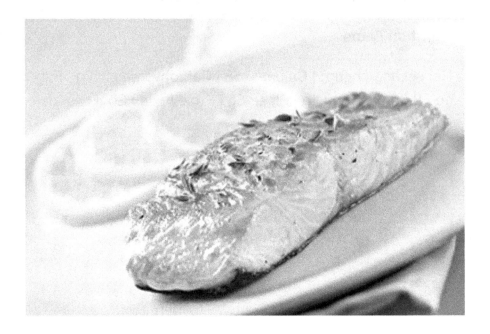

Preparation Time: 5 minutes

Cooking Time: 10-12 minutes

Yield: 2 servings

Ingredients

- 2 x 5 oz. pieces salmon with skin
- 1 tablespoon fresh tarragon leaves
- 1 tablespoon chives, chopped
- 2 teaspoons extra-virgin olive oil

Directions

1. Preheat oven to 425°F.

2. Rub the salmon with olive oil. Place the fish, skin side down, on a baking sheet lined with aluminum foil. Transfer baking sheet to the oven.
3. Bake the salmon for about 10-12 minutes or until cooked through. Once done, the salmon should flake easily with a fork.
4. Transfer salmon to a clean chopping board. Slice off the skin and transfer the salmon to a serving plate. You can discard the skin.
5. Before serving, sprinkle the salmon with herbs.

Nutrition Facts

Per serving (1 salmon fillet) | Calories: 207 | Carbohydrates: 3.08g | Fat: 8.72g | Saturated Fat: 1.67g | Fiber: 0.1g | Protein: 29.36g | Sodium: 113mg | Sugar: 0.03g

Citrusy Grilled Tilapia & Pineapple Salsa

Preparation Time: 10 minutes

Cooking Time: 10 minutes

Yield: 8 tilapia fillets and 2 cups of salsa

Ingredients

- 8 tilapia fillets (4 ounces each)
- 2 cups fresh pineapple, cubed
- 2 green onions, chopped
- ¼ cup fresh cilantro, minced
- ¼ cup green pepper, finely chopped
- 4 teaspoons lime juice, (plus 2 tablespoons) divided
- 1 tablespoon canola oil
- ⅛ teaspoon salt, (plus ¼ teaspoon) divided
- ⅛ teaspoon black pepper
- DASH cayenne pepper

Directions

1. For the salsa, combine the pineapple, green pepper, green onions, cilantro, and 4 teaspoons lime juice. Season with ⅛ teaspoon salt and cayenne pepper. Cool in the fridge until serving.
2. Mix the remaining lime juice and oil. Drizzle the mixture over the tilapia fillets then sprinkle with salt and pepper.

3. Spray the grill with a nonstick spray before laying the fillets. Cover and grill the tilapia over medium heat or until the fish easily flakes using a fork. Alternatively, you can broil the fish 4 inches from the heat for 2-3 minutes on each side. Serve with the salsa.

Nutrition Facts

Per serving (1 tilapia and ¼ cup salsa) | Calories: 131 | Carbohydrates: 6g | Fat: 3g | Saturated Fat: 1g | Fiber: 1g | Protein: 21g | Sodium: 152mg | Sugar: 4g

Chicken-Orange Heart-Friendly Tortilla

Preparation Time: 5 minutes

Cooking Time: 5-7 minutes

Yield: 4 servings

Ingredients

- 1 x 8 oz. chicken breast
- 1 large whole-wheat tortilla
- $\frac{2}{3}$ cup canned mandarin oranges, drained
- 4 large lettuce leaves, washed and patted dry
- $\frac{1}{2}$ cup celery, diced
- $\frac{1}{4}$ cup onion, minced
- 2 tablespoons low-sodium, low-calorie mayonnaise
- 1 teaspoon tamari sauce
- $\frac{1}{4}$ teaspoon garlic powder
- $\frac{1}{4}$ teaspoon black pepper

Directions

1. Place a nonstick pan over medium-high heat and cook the chicken breast until its internal temperature reaches 165°F. Remove from the heat and let cool. Once cool to the touch, cut it into half-inch cubes.
2. Mix the chicken, celery, onions, and oranges in a medium bowl. Add the tamari sauce, garlic,

mayonnaise, and pepper then mix until the chicken is evenly coated.

3. Place the tortilla on a large plate or cutting board. Cut it into quarters using a knife or kitchen scissors. Lay a lettuce leaf on each tortilla quarter, trimming off the excess, so it doesn't hang over the tortilla.

4. Spoon a quarter of the chicken mixture at the center of each lettuce leaf. Roll them up into a cone, with the two sides coming together and the curved edge forming the opening of the cone. Serve immediately.

Nutrition Facts

Per serving (¼ tortilla) | Calories: 166 | Carbohydrates: 10.64g | Fat: 7.66g | Saturated Fat: 2.25g | Fiber: 2g | Protein: 13.59g | Sodium: 193mg | Sugar: 3.96g

Quick & Easy Balsamic Chicken with Veggies

Preparation Time: 10 minutes

Cooking Time: 13 minutes

Yield: 4 servings

Ingredients

- 1¼ lbs. chicken breast tenderloins
- 1 lb. fresh asparagus, trimmed and chopped into 2-inch pieces
- 1½ cups carrots, cut into matchsticks
- 1 cup grape tomatoes, halved
- ¼ cup Italian salad dressing (plus 2 tablespoons), divided
- 3 tablespoons balsamic vinegar
- 1½ tablespoons honey
- ⅛ teaspoon crushed red pepper flakes
- 2 tablespoons olive oil
- ¼ teaspoon ground black pepper
- Pinch of salt

Directions

1. In a medium bowl, whisk the salad dressing, honey, balsamic vinegar, and red pepper flakes together then set aside.

2. Place a 12-inch skillet over medium-high heat and add oil. Meanwhile, rub the chicken with salt and pepper. Once the oil is hot, put the chicken into the skillet and cook about 6-7 minutes. Flip the chicken halfway through cooking time.
3. Once the chicken is thoroughly cooked, add half the dressing mixture and flip chicken to coat evenly.
4. Transfer the chicken to a large serving plate but leave the sauce in the skillet. Stir the carrots and asparagus into the sauce then continue to cook about 4 minutes, stirring frequently until the veggies are crisp and tender. Once done, transfer the veggies (together with the sauce) to the platter with chicken.
5. In the same skillet, add the remaining dressing mixture and cook, stirring constantly until it thickens. Return the chicken and the veggies to the skillet and toss to coat. Alternatively, pour the sauce over the chicken. Add tomatoes. Serve hot.

Nutrition Facts

Per serving (about 380g) | Calories: 342 | Carbohydrates: 20g | Fat: 14g | Saturated Fat: 2g | Fiber: 4g | Protein: 33g | Sodium: 351mg | Sugar: 15g

Baked Halibut and Tomato Salsa

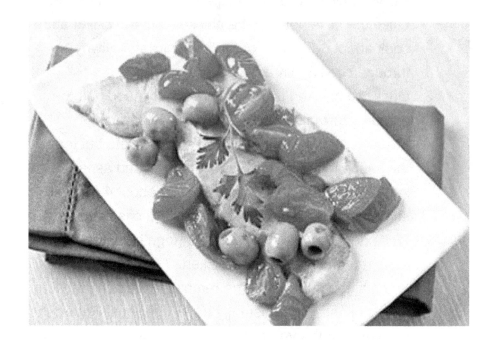

Preparation Time: 10 minutes

Cooking Time: 10-15 minutes

Yield: 4 servings

Ingredients

- 4 x 4 oz. halibut fillets
- 2 tomatoes, diced
- 2 tablespoons fresh basil, chopped
- 1 tablespoon garlic, minced
- 2 teaspoons extra-virgin olive oil
- 1 teaspoon fresh oregano, chopped

Directions

1. Preheat the oven to 350°F and lightly grease a 9x13-inch baking pan with a nonstick cooking spray.
2. Combine the basil, tomato, garlic, and oregano in a small bowl. Add the olive oil and toss, making sure everything is coated.
3. Lay the halibut fillets in the baking pan and spoon tomato mixture over them. Put into the oven and bake about 10-15 minutes or until the fish is completely opaque. Use a knife to check the thickest part of each fillet.
4. Once done, transfer to serving plates and serve with vegetables.

Nutrition Facts

Per serving (1 halibut fillet) | Calories: 128 | Carbohydrates: 3g | Fat: 4g | Saturated Fat: 1g | Fiber: 1g | Protein: 22g | Sodium: 81mg | Sugar: 0g

Nutty Spinach & Blue Cheese Salad

Preparation Time: 15 minutes

Yield: 12 servings

Ingredients

For the salad:

- 2 lbs. spinach (or 3 x 10-oz packages), roughly chopped
- ¼ cup blue cheese crumbles
- ¼ cup walnuts, chopped
- ½ cup red onion, sliced
- 1½ cups grape tomatoes
- 1½ cups cucumbers, sliced

For the dressing:

- 2 tablespoons balsamic vinegar
- 1 tablespoon plain low-fat yogurt
- 1 tablespoon maple syrup
- 4 teaspoons olive oil
- ¼ teaspoon nutmeg

Directions

1. For the dressing, process all ingredients in a food processor or blender. Chill the dressing with the serving plate (or plates) you're going to use for lunch.
2. In a salad bowl, toss the spinach with the dressing to coat. Measure 2 cups and place onto chilled plates. Top with vegetables, blue cheese crumbles, and walnuts then serve immediately.

Nutrition Facts

Per serving (2½ cups) | Calories: 70 | Carbohydrates: 7g | Fat: 4g | Saturated Fat: 1g | Fiber: 2g | Protein: 4g | Sodium: 95mg | Sugar: 1g

Cheesy Chicken & Spinach Tortilla Casserole

Preparation Time: 25 minutes

Cooking Time: 50 minutes

Yield: 9 servings

Ingredients

- 1 lb. boneless, skinless chicken breasts, trimmed
- 12 corn tortillas, halved
- 4 oz. goat cheese
- 8 oz. mushrooms, sliced
- 4 cups baby spinach
- 2 cups low-fat milk
- ¼ cup pickled jalapeños, chopped
- ⅓ cup Mexican cheese blend, shredded
- ⅓ cup green salsa
- 2 tablespoons extra-virgin olive oil
- 3 cloves garlic, sliced
- 1 medium leek (light green and white only), halved and sliced
- 1 tablespoon cornstarch
- ¼ teaspoon salt
- ¼ teaspoon ground pepper

Directions

1. Preheat oven to 400°F and grease a 9x13-inch baking dish with a nonstick cooking spray.
2. Place the chicken in a medium saucepan and add enough water to cover it by 1 inch. Turn heat to medium heat and bring it to a boil. Adjust the heat to low and cover the saucepan with the lid. Bring it to a gentle simmer for about 10-12 minutes or until the chicken is completely cooked.
3. Transfer the chicken to a clean chopping board and shred it using two forks.
4. Place a large pot over medium-high heat and add oil. Sauté the garlic, leeks, and mushrooms. Cook and occasionally stir for about 4 minutes or until the leek is tender and starting to brown.
5. Mix the cornstarch and milk in a small bowl and add into the pot. Continue to cook about $3\frac{1}{2}$ minutes, stirring constantly until the mixture thickens.
6. Add the goat cheese, jalapeños, and spinach. Season with salt and pepper. Cook another 2 minutes or until the spinach wilts and the cheese melts. Add the shredded chicken and turn off the heat.
7. Assemble 6 tortilla halves at the bottom of the baking dish. Measure $1\frac{1}{2}$ cups of chicken mixture and spread over the tortillas. Repeat these steps until the tortillas and spread are finished, with the tortillas as the top layer.
8. Spread the green salsa on top and top with shredded Mexican cheese.

9. Bake about 20-25 minutes or until bubbly. Carefully remove the casserole from the oven and allow to stand for about 10 minutes before serving.

Nutrition Facts

Per serving (⅔ cup) | Calories: 255 | Carbohydrates: 22g | Fat: 10g | Saturated Fat: 4g | Fiber: 3g | Protein: 20g | Sodium: 281mg | Sugar: 4g

Autumn-Flavored Spinach Salad

Preparation Time: 30-35 minutes

Yield: 8 servings

Ingredients

- 8 cups fresh baby spinach leaves, stemmed
- 2 pears (ripe and unpeeled), quartered lengthwise, cored, and cut into long, thin slices
- ⅓ cup sweetened dried cranberries
- ⅔ cup hazelnuts, toasted and chopped
- 1 cup red onion, thinly sliced

For the dressing:

- ½ cup extra-virgin olive oil
- 2 tablespoons balsamic vinegar
- 2 teaspoons whole-grain mustard
- 1 teaspoon brown sugar
- 1 teaspoon kosher or sea salt
- Freshly ground pepper

Directions

1. Fill a medium bowl with cold water then add the onions. Set aside for about 30 minutes. This process allows the onion to crisp and removes the raw taste. Drain the water and dry with paper towels.

2. Meanwhile, for the dressing, combine the ingredients in a small mason jar with a tight-fitting lid. Make sure to cover the jar tightly before shaking it to mix all ingredients.
3. Place the cranberries in a small bowl and add 2 tablespoons of dressing. Toss to soften the fruit. Let stand approximately 15 minutes or until the salad is ready to serve.
4. For the salad, combine the pears, spinach, and onions in a large bowl. Shake the jar of dressing before pouring it over the salad. Toss to coat.
5. Serve in a large salad bowl or divide among 8 serving plates. Top each with cranberries and hazelnuts then serve.

Nutrition Facts

Per serving ($\frac{1}{2}$ cup) | Calories: 252 | Carbohydrates: 17g | Fat: 21g | Saturated Fat: 2g | Fiber: 3g | Protein: 2g | Sodium: 250mg | Sugar: 9.6g

Teriyaki Salmon & Broccoli

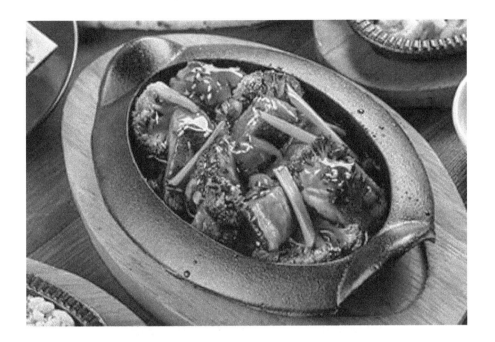

Preparation Time: 15 minutes

Cooking Time: 18 minutes

Yield: 4 servings

Ingredients

- 4 x 4-oz salmon fillets
- 1½ lbs. broccoli head, cut into florets, stalks peeled and cut in ¼ inch coins
- ½ cup almonds, sliced
- 4 scallions, trimmed and thinly sliced
- 2 cloves garlic, minced

- 2 tablespoons honey
- 2 tablespoons low-sodium teriyaki sauce
- 1 tablespoon rice wine vinegar
- 2 teaspoons cornstarch
- ¼ cup water

Directions

1. Combine the teriyaki sauce, honey, garlic, scallions, and vinegar in a small bowl. Divide the mixture in half and set aside.
2. Adjust the top oven rack 6 inches from the heat. Preheat the broiler and prepare the baking sheet by lining it with foil.
3. Next, place a large nonstick skillet over medium-high heat. Once it's hot, toast the almonds for about 6 minutes. Without turning off the heat, transfer the almonds to a bowl and wipe the skillet with a paper towel.
4. Put ¼ cup of water in the skillet and reduce the heat to medium-low. Add the broccoli and cover the skillet with a lid. Cook about 7-8 minutes until tender and the color turns bright green.
5. Put the salmon into the baking sheet and brush it with half the teriyaki mixture. Broil the fish about 5-8 minutes or until the internal temperature reaches 120°F.
6. Stir the cornstarch into the remaining half teriyaki mixture and pour into the skillet. Bring to a simmer and cook about 4 minutes, stirring constantly until it reaches the consistency of a glaze. Add the almonds.

7. Transfer salmon and broccoli teriyaki mixture onto serving plates.

Nutrition Facts

Per serving (1 salmon fillet and ¼ portion of broccoli) | Calories: 332 | Carbohydrates: 25g | Fat: 14g | Saturated Fat: 2g | Fiber: 6g | Protein: 30g | Sodium: 239mg | Sugar: 2g

Healthy Pomegranate & Ricotta Bruschetta

Preparation Time: 15 minutes

Cooking Time: 8 minutes

Yield: 2 servings

Ingredients

- 1 cup low-fat ricotta cheese
- ½ cup pomegranate arils
- 6 slices whole-grain nut bread
- ½ teaspoon lemon zest
- 2 teaspoons thyme, fresh
- ¼ teaspoon sea salt

Directions

- Preheat the oven to 425°F and arrange the bread slices on a large baking sheet. Bake them for about 8 minutes or until lightly roasted.
- Combine the ricotta and lemon zest in a small bowl.
- Top each toast with ricotta mixture then sprinkle with pomegranate arils and thyme.

Nutrition Facts

Per serving (3 bruschetta) | Calories: 257 | Carbohydrates: 39g | Fat: 6g | Saturated Fat: 2g | Fiber: 4g | Protein: 13g | Sodium: 383mg | Sugar: 11g

Dinner

DASH Steak Salad with Roasted Corn Dressing

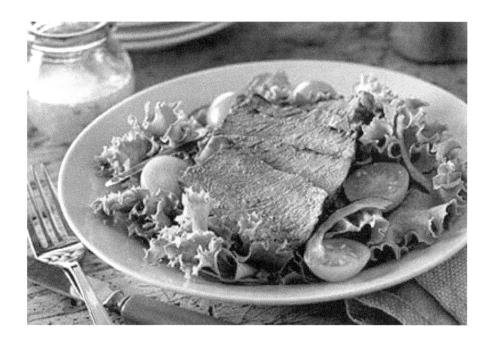

Preparation Time: 10 minutes

Cooking Time: 20 minutes

Yield: 6 servings

Ingredients

- ¾ lb. flank steak
- 1½ cups black beans, cooked but without added salt
- 3 cups fresh corn kernels (about 4-5 ears of corn)

- 1 large head (about 6 cups) romaine lettuce, trimmed and torn into bite-sized pieces
- 4 cups cherry tomatoes, halved
- ¾ cup red onion, thinly sliced
- ¼ cup fresh cilantro (or fresh coriander), chopped
- ½ cup water
- 2 tablespoons fresh lime juice
- 2 tablespoons red bell pepper, chopped
- 2 tablespoons extra-virgin olive oil
- 2 teaspoons dried oregano
- 1 tablespoon ground cumin
- ½ teaspoon salt, divided
- ½ teaspoon freshly ground black pepper, divided
- ¼ teaspoon red pepper flakes

Directions

1. Put a heavy nonstick skillet over medium-high heat. Once hot, add the corn and cook about 4-5 minutes or until the kernels begin to brown then turn off the heat.
2. For the dressing, combine 1 cup of roasted corn kernels, bell pepper, water, and lime juice in a blender or food processor. Process the ingredients until pureed. Add the olive oil, cilantro, ¼ teaspoon salt, and ¼ teaspoon ground black pepper. Pulse again before transferring to a mason jar or a small bowl.

3. Spritz your grill rack or broiler pan with a nonstick cooking spray. Position the cooking rack 4 to 6 inches from the heat source.
4. Incorporate the red pepper flakes, cumin, oregano, plus the remaining salt and pepper in a small bowl. Rub the steak on both sides with this mixture.
5. Put the steak on the rack or pan. Grill or broil the steak about 4-5 minutes on each side. To check, use a meat thermometer (160°F for medium doneness) or cut into the center. Let stand 5 minutes and cut across the grain, making 2-inch long meat slices.
6. Combine the black beans, remaining roasted corn, lettuce, tomatoes, and onion in a large salad bowl. Add the dressing and toss gently to coat.
7. Divide the salad among serving plates and top with steak slices to serve.

Nutrition Facts

Per serving (2 ounces of steak and 2½ cups salad) | Calories: 295 | Carbohydrates: 37g | Fat: 9g | Saturated Fat: 2g | Fiber: 9g | Protein: 21g | Sodium: 249mg | Sugar: 7g

Baked Broccoli & Cauliflower with Piquant Yogurt Sauce

Preparation Time: 15 minutes

Cooking Time: 25-27 minutes

Yield: 8 servings

Ingredients

- 8 cups broccoli florets
- 8 cups cauliflower florets
- ⅓ cup plain, non-fat yogurt
- ¼ cup olive oil
- 2 cloves garlic, sliced
- ½ teaspoon hot paprika
- ½ teaspoon smoked paprika
- ½ teaspoon salt
- ⅛ teaspoon black pepper

Directions

1. Preheat oven to 400°F.
2. Meanwhile, combine the broccoli, cauliflower, black pepper, ½ teaspoon of salt, and 3 tablespoons olive oil in a large bowl then toss to combine.
3. Divide the broccoli-cauliflower mixture between 2 rimmed baking sheets, arranging them in one layer.

Bake at 400°F for about 15 minutes; stir and bake an additional 10 minutes.

4. Meanwhile, place a small saucepan over medium heat and add 1 tablespoon olive oil. When the oil is hot enough, add garlic and both types of paprika; cook 2 minutes.

5. Add the seasoned garlic to the yogurt. Drizzle over the baked veggies and serve.

Nutrition Facts

Per serving (about ¾ cup) | Calories: 116 | Carbohydrates: 11g | Fat: 7g | Saturated Fat: 1g | Fiber: 4g |Protein:4g | Sodium: 240mg | Sugar: 2g

Healthy Ziti & Meatballs

Preparation Time: 30 minutes

Cooking Time: 12 minutes

Yield: 8 servings

Ingredients

- 1 lb. ground sirloin
- 1 x 16-oz box ziti
- 8 oz. mushrooms, trimmed, cleaned and grated
- 5 oz. baby kale, chopped
- ½ cup grated parmesan, divided
- ½ cup Italian seasoned dry bread crumbs
- ½ cup low-sodium chicken broth
- 1 large egg
- 2 tablespoons canola oil
- 3 cloves garlic, sliced
- ½ teaspoon crushed red pepper flakes
- ½ teaspoon salt, divided
- ½ teaspoon black pepper, divided

Directions

1. Mix the sirloin, mushroom, egg, and ¼ cup Parmesan, and bread crumbs. Season with ¼ teaspoon each of

pepper and salt. With wet hands, make ¾-1-inch balls (approximately 54 pieces).

2. Place a large pot of salted water over medium-high heat and bring to a boil. Once boiling, add the ziti and cook 10 minutes. Turn off the heat; reserve half a cup of pasta water and drain.

3. Heat 1 tablespoon oil in a large nonstick skillet placed over medium-high heat. Add half the meatballs and cook about 4 minutes, turning each until browned all over. Transfer the first batch to a large platter. Repeat this step for the remaining meatballs. When done, remove the meatballs from the skillet.

4. Adjust the heat to medium, add the garlic, kale, and red pepper flakes in the same skillet; cook for 2 minutes. Add the reserved pasta water, chicken broth plus the remaining salt and pepper. Cook 2 minutes more and add the ziti.

5. Combine the pasta mixture and meatballs in a large bowl. Add the remaining quarter cup Parmesan; toss to combine and serve.

Nutrition Facts

Per serving (⅛ of the recipe) | Calories: 497 | Carbohydrates: 66g | Fat: 12g | Saturated Fat: 3g | Fiber: 4g | Protein: 31g | Sodium: 517mg | Sugar: 4g

Spiced Beef Kebabs

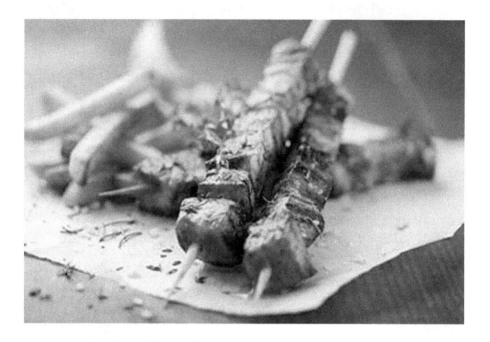

Preparation Time: 2 hours and 15 minutes

Cooking Time: 30 minutes

Yield: 6 servings

Ingredients

- 2 lbs. sirloin flap steak or flatiron steak, cut into 1½-inch pieces
- 2 cloves garlic, minced
- ¼ cup olive oil
- 2 tablespoons oregano, finely chopped
- 2 teaspoons ground cumin

- 1 teaspoon ground coriander
- ¼ teaspoon cayenne
- Pinch of salt

Directions

1. Soak twelve 12-inch wooden skewers in water for about 30 minutes.
2. Incorporate the garlic, oregano, oil, salt, and the spices in a bowl. Add the beef then keep chilled and marinate for at least 2 hours.
3. After 2 hours, prepare the grill, setting it over medium-hot charcoal (or high heat for gas).
4. Meanwhile, skewer about 4 pieces of beef, leaving small spaces in between. Put each on a tray.
5. Brush the rack with oil or spray it with a nonstick cooking spray. Grill the beef for about 4-5 minutes, turning occasionally to make sure they're cooked thoroughly (if you're using a gas grill, cover the beef).

Nutrition Facts

Per serving (2 kebobs) | Calories: 385 | Carbohydrates: 2g | Fat: 29g | Saturated Fat: 9g |Fiber: 1g

Orange, Beet & Ricotta Salad

Preparation Time: 5-8 minutes

Cooking Time: 18-20 minutes

Yield: 4 servings

Ingredients

- 2 navel oranges
- 1½ lbs. medium beets, peeled and cut into wedges
- ¼ cup part-skim ricotta cheese
- 2 cups baby arugula
- 1½ tablespoons extra-virgin olive oil
- Pinch of salt
- Pinch of pepper
- Caraway seeds

Directions

1. Put the beets in a large saucepan and cover with water. Bring to a boil then lower the heat, letting it simmer about 15 minutes until the beets are tender. Drain the water and set aside.
2. Grate about 2 teaspoons of orange zest. Peel the oranges and divide into segments. Make 2 tablespoons orange juice from some of the segments. Combine the juice, zest, olive oil, salt and pepper in a bowl.

3. Put half a cup of arugula on each of the 4 serving plates. Divide the beets and orange segments among 4 plates. Drizzle each portion with the dressing and top with 1 tbsp. ricotta. Garnish with caraway seeds before serving.

Nutrition Facts

Per serving (1¼ cups) | Calories: 132 | Carbohydrates: 15g | Fat: 7g | Saturated Fat: 2g | Fiber: 3g | Protein: 4g | Sodium: 88mg | Sugar: 9.8g

Tomato & Corn Cheese Tortellini

Preparation Time: 10 minutes

Cooking Time: 10-12 minutes

Yield: 4 servings

Ingredients

- 1 x 9 oz. package cheese tortellini, refrigerated
- 2 cups cherry tomatoes, quartered
- 3⅓ cups fresh (or frozen) corn kernels
- ¼ cup fresh basil, minced
- 2 green onions, thinly sliced
- 4 teaspoons olive oil
- 2 tablespoons grated parmesan cheese
- ¼ teaspoon garlic powder
- ⅛ teaspoon black pepper

Directions

1. Place a pot filled with water over medium-high heat and cook the tortellini as per package instructions. Add the corn kernels in the last 5 minutes of cooking. Drain and transfer to a large bowl.
2. Add the rest of the ingredients to the bowl and mix (or toss) to coat.

Nutrition Facts

Per serving (1¾ cups) | Calories: 366 | Carbohydrates: 57g |
Fat: 12g | Saturated Fat: 4g | Fiber: 5g | Protein: 14g | Sodium:
286mg | Sugar: 6g

Apricot-Glazed Balsamic Turkey

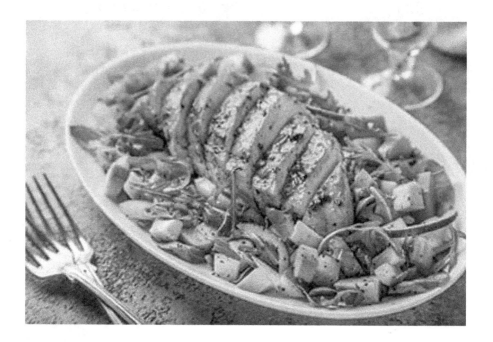

Preparation Time: 10 minutes

Cooking Time: 1½-2 hours

Yield: 15 servings

Ingredients

- 1 x 5 lbs. bone-in turkey breast
- ½ cup apricot preserves
- ¼ cup balsamic vinegar
- ¼ teaspoon black pepper
- DASH salt

Directions

1. Preheat oven to 325°F. Mix the apricots, vinegar, salt, and pepper in a small bowl. Put the turkey breast on a rack placed in a large, shallow roasting pan.
2. Bake without a cover for 1½-2 hours, basting it with apricot glaze every 30 minutes. If the turkey browns easily, loosely cover it with foil.
3. Once done, cover the turkey and let stand about 15 minutes before slicing.

Nutrition Facts

Per serving (4 ounces cooked turkey) | Calories: 236 | Carbohydrates: 8g | Fat: 8g | Saturated Fat: 2g | Fiber: 0g | Protein: 32g | Sodium: 84mg | Sugar: 5g

Simple DASH Strawberry Salad

Preparation Time: 15 minutes

Yield: 6 servings

Ingredients

- 1 head romaine lettuce, torn into bite-size pieces
- 1 cup fresh strawberries, sliced
- ½ cup pecans, toasted
- ¼ cup red bell pepper, chopped
- ½ cup fat-free creamy salad dressing
- ¼ cup milk
- ¼ cup white sugar
- ⅛ cup distilled white vinegar
- 1 tablespoon poppy seeds
- ½ red onion, sliced

Directions

- Mix the milk, sugar, salad dressing, poppy seeds, and vinegar in a small bowl. Chill in the fridge until ready to use.
- In a salad bowl, combine the strawberries, lettuce, red bell pepper, onion, and pecans. Drizzle with dressing and toss to coat before serving.

Nutrition Facts

Per serving (¾ cup) | Calories: 151 | Carbohydrates: 18.8g | Fat: 8.4g | Saturated Fat: 1g | Fiber: 3.4g | Protein: 2.5g | Sodium: 177mg | Sugar: 14g

Quick & Easy Avocado Salad

Preparation Time: 10 minutes

Yield: 6 servings

Ingredients

- 2 avocados
- 1 large ripe tomato, chopped
- 1 green bell pepper, chopped
- 1 sweet onion, chopped
- ¼ cup fresh cilantro, chopped
- ½ lime, juiced
- Pinch of salt
- ¼ teaspoon black pepper

Directions

1. Slice the avocado in half, remove the seed, and scoop the thin membrane in the hole where the seed had been. Make slices across the avocado halves, forming grids. Carefully scoop the avocado cubes and transfer to a salad bowl.
2. Add the rest of the ingredients to the bowl and toss. Serve chilled or as is.

Nutrition Facts

Per serving (½ cup) | Calories: 126 | Carbohydrates: 10.2g | Fat: 10g | Saturated Fat: 1g | Fiber: 5.7g | Protein: 2.1g | Sodium: 9mg | Sugar: 3g

Wholesome Vegetable Pizza

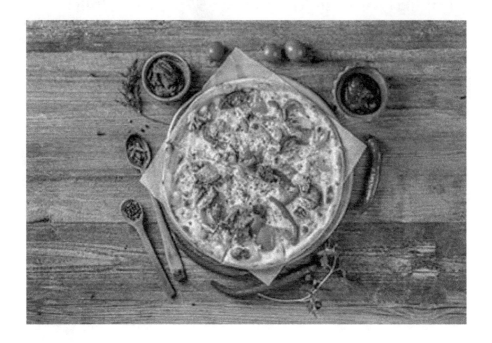

Preparation Time: 40 minutes (plus rising)

Cooking Time: 20 minutes

Yield: 2 pizzas (12 slices total)

Ingredients

For the dough:

- ½ cup whole-wheat flour
- 2½ cups all-purpose flour
- 2 x 0.25-oz package quick-rise yeast
- 1 cup water
- 2 tablespoons olive oil

- 1 teaspoon garlic powder
- ½ teaspoon salt

For the sauce:

- 1 x 14.5 oz. can diced tomatoes, not drained
- 1 tablespoon fresh parsley, minced
- 1½ teaspoons sugar
- 1½ teaspoons Italian seasoning
- 1½ teaspoons dried basil
- ½ teaspoon garlic powder
- ¼ teaspoon pepper

For the toppings:

- 1¼ cups part-skim mozzarella cheese, shredded
- 1 cup zucchini, chopped
- 1 cup fresh mushrooms, sliced
- ½ cup green or red pepper, chopped
- ¼ cup onion, chopped
- 1 teaspoon olive oil

Directions

1. For the dough, combine the whole-wheat flour, yeast, garlic powder, salt, and 1 cup all-purpose flour. Place a small saucepan over medium-high heat. Heat the water with oil to 120°F-130°F then add to dry ingredients.

Using a stand mixer, beat the mixture for about 3 minutes until soft dough is formed.

2. Sprinkle flour on a clean surface. Knead the dough for 5 minutes or until elastic and smooth. Grease a bowl, put the dough inside, and grease the exposed part of the dough with oil. Cover with a clean kitchen towel or plastic wrap and let it rise in a warm place for about 30 minutes or until it's doubled in size.

3. Meanwhile, place a small saucepan over medium heat. Add all the sauce ingredients and bring to a boil. Reduce the heat, letting it simmer uncovered for 15-18 minutes. Stir occasionally to avoid burning. Turn off the heat once a slightly thick consistency is achieved.

4. Preheat the oven to 400°F and punch down the dough. Sprinkle flour on a clean surface, divide the dough in half, and roll each half into a 12-inch round. Place on two greased 12-inch pizza pans and prick the dough with a fork. Bake 8-10 minutes or until lightly browned.

5. For the toppings, place a skillet over medium-high heat and sauté the vegetables until the zucchini is crisp-tender.

6. To assemble, smear the crusts with sauce then garnish with vegetables and cheese. Bring back to the oven and bake 12-15 minutes or until the cheese has melted.

Nutrition Facts

Per serving (1 slice) | Calories: 190 | Carbohydrates: 28g | Fat: 6g | Saturated Fat: 2g | Fiber: 3g | Protein: 7g | Sodium: 234mg | Sugar: 3g

Lemony and Peppery Tuna Steak

Preparation Time: 15-18 minutes

Cooking Time: 25 minutes

Yield: 6 servings

Ingredients

- 6 x 8 oz. tuna steaks, 1-inch thick
- ¼ cup whole black peppercorns
- 2 tablespoons fresh lemon juice
- 2 tablespoons extra-virgin olive oil
- DASH of salt
- DASH of pepper

Directions

1. Put the tuna in a large bowl. Add the lemon juice, salt, pepper, and oil. Make sure all sides of tuna are coated with the marinade. Let it stand about 15-20 minutes, turning once halfway through the marinating period.
2. Put the peppercorns in a clean cloth or thick plastic bag. Crush them using a mortar and pestle (or using a small mallet) and transfer to a large plate.
3. Dip the edges of the tuna steak into the crushed peppercorns.
4. Preheat a nonstick skillet over medium heat. Working in batches, sear the tuna steaks for about 4 minutes per

side. If necessary, pour 2-3 tablespoons of the marinade to the skillet to prevent sticking. Serve.

Nutrition Facts

Per serving (1 tuna steak) | Calories: 345 | Carbohydrates: 1.2g | Fat: 9.3g | Saturated Fat: 0.7g | Fiber: 0.4g | Protein: 63.7g | Sodium: 29mg |Sugar: 0.1g

DASH Chicken Chili

Preparation Time: 5-8 minutes

Cooking Time: 20 minutes

Yield: 8 servings

Ingredients

- 1 x 10 oz. can white chunk chicken
- 1 x 14.5 oz. can low-sodium diced tomatoes
- 2 x 15 oz. can low-sodium white beans, drained
- 4 cups low-sodium chicken broth
- 1 medium red pepper, chopped
- 1 medium onion, chopped
- ½ medium green pepper, chopped
- 2 cloves garlic, minced
- 8 tablespoons reduced-fat Monterey Jack cheese, shredded
- 3 tablespoons fresh cilantro, chopped
- 2 teaspoons chili powder
- 1 teaspoon ground cumin
- 1 teaspoon dried oregano
- Cayenne pepper

Directions

1. Place the chicken, broth, tomatoes, and beans in a large soup pot. Cover the pot with a lid and let simmer over medium heat.

2. Spritz a nonstick skillet with cooking spray and place over medium-high heat. Sauté the onions, garlic, and peppers about 3-5 minutes or until the veggies are tender.
3. Add the sautéed vegetables into the pot then stir in the spices. Simmer another 10 minutes or until the veggies are soft.
4. Divide among serving bowls. Top with 1 tablespoon cheese and cilantro.

Nutrition Facts

Per serving (1½ cups) | Calories: 212 | Carbohydrates: 25g | Fat: 4g | Saturated Fat: 1.5g | Fiber: 6g | Protein: 19g | Sodium: 241mg | Sugar: 4g

Summer Salad with Grilled Shrimp

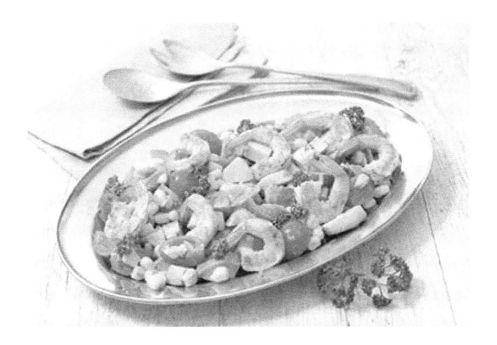

Preparation Time: 20 minutes

Cooking Time: 8-10 minutes

Yield: 4 servings

Ingredients

- 1 lb. (around 31-40 pieces) raw shrimp peeled and deveined
- 4 medium ears sweet corn, husked
- 1 medium ripe avocado, peeled and chopped
- 1½ cups cherry tomatoes, halved
- ½ cup packed fresh basil leaves

- ¼ cup olive oil
- ½ teaspoon salt, divided
- ⅛ teaspoon black pepper

Directions

1. Prepare the wooden skewers by soaking them in water for 30 minutes.
2. Bring a pot of water to a boil and cook the corn about 5 minutes or until tender. Drain and let cool.
3. Blend the basil, oil, and ¼ teaspoon salt in a blender or food processor.
4. Cut corn from the cob and transfer to a bowl. Add in the tomatoes then season with salt and pepper. Mix in the avocado and 2 tablespoons basil mixture. Gently toss to combine.
5. Thread the shrimp onto skewers and brush with the basil mixture leftover. Place the skewers on the grill. Cover and cook over medium heat for 2-4 minutes on each side or until shrimp are pink and opaque. Remove shrimp from skewers and divide among serving plates. Serve with the prepared salad on the side.

Nutrition Facts

Per serving (1 cup) | Calories: 371 | Carbohydrates: 25g | Fat: 22g | Saturated Fat: 3g | Fiber: 5g | Protein: 23g | Sodium: 450mg | Sugar: 8g

Ultimate DASH Burger

Preparation Time: 15 minutes

Cooking Time: 8-15 minutes

Yield: 4 servings

Ingredients

- 4 whole-wheat or multigrain hamburger buns, split
- 1 lb. lean ground turkey
- ¼ cup fresh basil, chopped
- 3 tablespoons mesquite smoke-flavored barbecue sauce
- 2 tablespoons quick-cooking oats or oat bran
- 1 clove garlic, minced
- ¼ teaspoon garlic salt
- ⅛ teaspoon black pepper

For the toppings (optional):

- Provolone cheese, sliced
- Red onion slices
- Sliced tomato
- Fresh basil leaves

Directions

1. Combine the garlic, basil, oats, barbecue sauce, garlic salt, and pepper in a large bowl. Gently mix in the

turkey, being careful not to overmix everything. Divide the mixture into four equal portions and shape each into half-inch patties.

2. Lightly grease a grill rack and grill burgers, covered, over medium heat until center is no longer pink and a food thermometer reads 165°F, approximately 5-7 minutes per side.
3. Grill buns over medium heat (with the cut-side down) for 30-60 seconds or until toasted.
4. Serve the burgers with toppings if desired.

Note: Nutritional info does not include toppings.

Nutrition Facts

Per serving (1 burger) | Calories: 315 | Carbohydrates: 29g | Fat: 11g | Saturated Fat: 3g | Fiber: 4g | Protein: 27g | Sodium: 482mg | Sugar: 8g

Bonus DASH recipes

Breakfast Recipes

Granola Yogurt Breakfast Bowl

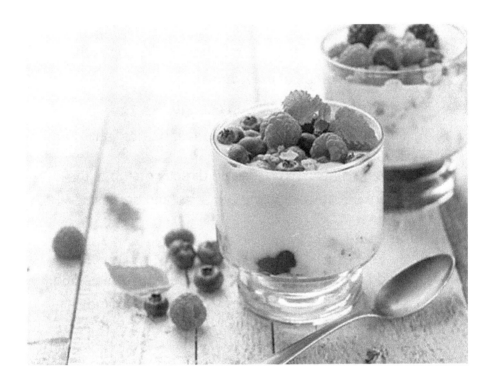

Preparation Time: 5 minutes

Yield: 1 serving

Ingredients

- ¾ cup unsweetened coconut yogurt

- ½ cup berries
- 1 small banana, sliced
- ⅓ cup granola
- Pure maple syrup(to taste, optional)*

Directions

1. Scoop ½ cup of yogurt into a bowl.
2. Top with half of the sliced bananas, ¼ cup of the berries, and half of the granola.
3. Add the remaining ¼ cup of yogurt.
4. Then top with remaining bananas, berries, and granola.

Note: If using maple syrup, drizzle directly on top of the yogurt layers before adding the bananas and berries.

Nutrition Facts

Per serving | Calories: 402 | Fat: 15g | Carbohydrates: 66g | Fiber: 11g | Sugars: 29g | Protein: 7g | Sodium: 57mg

No-Bake Yogurt and Berry Tart

Preparation Time: 30 minutes

Cooking Time: 0 minutes

Yield: 6 servings

Ingredients

For the crust:

- 2 cups raw pecans
- 10 Medjool dates, soaked in warm water for 10minutes and pitted
- ¼ teaspoon fine sea salt

For the filling:

- 1½ cups plain Greek yogurt
- ½ cup raspberries or blueberries (or more – I used a 6-ounce container)
- 4 strawberries, hulled and thinly sliced
- 2 tablespoons honey

Directions

1. In a food processor, pulse the pecans until ground into a semi-fine meal.
2. Add the dates and pulse until a sticky dough is formed.

3. Press dough evenly onto bottom and up sides of 9 to 9 ½-inch tart pan with a removable bottom.
4. Let the crust set in the freezer for 10 minutes.
5. Remove the crust from the freezer. Carefully remove the tart from the pan (leave it resting on the round base) and slide it onto a round serving platter.
6. Spoon the yogurt into the crust and smooth it out with a rubber spatula.
7. Decorate with the berries and drizzle with honey.
8. Slice and enjoy!

Nutrition Facts

Per serving (1 slice made with low fat Greek yogurt) | Calories: 403 | Fat: 24.8g | Carbohydrates: 44.1g | Fiber: 6.7g |Sugars: 36.2g | Protein: 8.8g | Sodium: 110.7mg

Pumpkin Spice Protein Pancakes

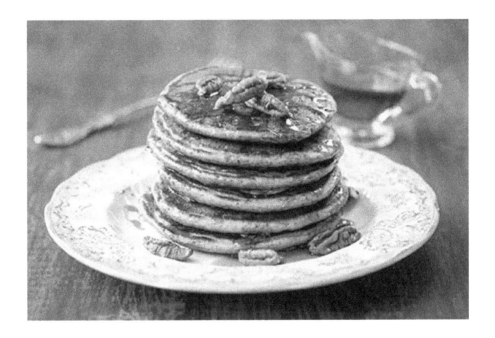

Preparation Time: 10 minutes

Cooking Time: 20 minutes

Yield: 8 pancakes

Ingredients

- 1 cup pumpkin puree
- 2 cups vanilla protein powder (I used whey protein)
- 2-3 tablespoons butter, for frying
- 4 egg whites

- 1 teaspoon pumpkin spice (or a mix of cinnamon, nutmeg and ginger)
- 1 teaspoon baking powder

Topping ideas:

- Shredded coconut
- Almond butter
- Pumpkin seeds
- Chopped walnuts or pecans

Directions

1. In a large bowl, mix all ingredients for pancakes until just combined.
2. Place the large non-stick frying pan over medium heat and add butter. Let the butter melt completely.
3. The pan needs to be hot enough to add pancake batter. Test it by putting a drop of batter in the pan. If it sizzles, it's hot enough.
4. Add pancake batter using a large ladle scoop, cooking four pancakes at a time and flipping once the bottom starts to form, about 5 minutes.
5. Serve the pancakes with any of the optional toppings. *

*Note: Nutritional info does not include toppings, such as shredded coconut, almond butter etc.

Nutrition Facts

Per serving (2 pancakes) | Calories: 182 | Fat: 8g | Carbohydrates: 10g | Fiber: 2g | Sugars: 4g | Protein: 22g | Sodium: 212mg

Berry Breakfast Toast

Preparation Time: 5 minutes

Cooking Time: 1-2 minutes

Yield: 1 serving

Ingredients

- 1 slice whole-grain bread
- 2 tablespoons mascarpone cheese
- ¼ cup berries, such as raspberries, blueberries and/or chopped strawberries
- 1 teaspoon mint leaves

Directions

1. In a toaster oven or under the broiler, lightly toast bread on both sides.
2. Spread toast with mascarpone. Top with berries and sprinkle with mint leaves.

Nutrition Facts

Per serving (1 slice) | Calories: 326 | Fat: 27g | Carbohydrates: 15g | Fiber: 4g | Sugars: 3g | Protein: 8g | Sodium: 130mg

Blueberry Banana Smoothie

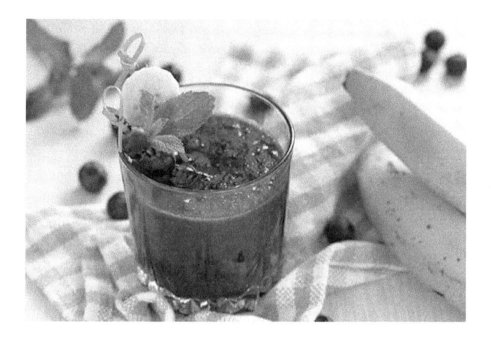

Preparation Time: 5 minutes

Cook Time: 0 minutes

Yield: 2 smoothies

Ingredients

- 1½ cup frozen bananas (I freeze my bananas in ½-inch slices)
- 1½ cups frozen blueberries
- 1½ cups to 2 cups unsweetened vanilla almond milk or water
- ¼ cup almond butter

- Optional nutrition boosters: ¼ cup old-fashioned oats and/or 2 tablespoons flax seed*

Directions

1. Place all ingredients in a blender.
2. Blend starting on low speed and increasing to high for 30-60 seconds or until the mixture is smooth and creamy.
3. Pour into cups and serve immediately.

*Note: Nutrition Information does not include optional add-ins (oats or flax seeds)

Nutrition Facts

Per serving (1 smoothie) | Calories: 386 | Fat: 21g | Carbohydrates: 47.1g | Fiber: 9.3g | Sugars: 25g | Protein: 9.6g | Sodium: 167mg

Fruit & Yogurt Quinoa Bowl

Preparation Time: 5 minutes

Cooking Time: 0 minutes

Yield: 2 servings

Ingredients

- 1 cup cooked quinoa, still warm
- 2 tablespoons coconut milk
- 2 tablespoons maple syrup+ more for drizzling
- 1 teaspoon cinnamon
- 1 cup non-dairy yogurt
- 1 medium peach, pit removed and cut into chunks
- 1 cup strawberries, stems removed and chopped
- ¼ cup chopped almonds
- 2 tablespoons hemp seeds

Directions

1. Add cooked quinoa, 2 tablespoons maple syrup, coconut milk and cinnamon to a small bowl. Stir to combine.
2. Divide evenly between two bowls. Top each bowl with yogurt, peach, and strawberries. Scatter the almonds and hemp seeds over top.
3. Drizzle with remaining maple syrup and enjoy!

Nutrition Facts

Per serving (½ of recipe) | Calories: 514 | Fat: 22g |
Carbohydrates: 63g | Fiber: 8g | Sugars: 29g | Protein: 17g |
Sodium: 95mg

Asparagus Frittata

Preparation Time: 15 minutes

Cooking Time: 25-35 minutes

Yield: 8 slices

Ingredients

- 1 bunch asparagus
- 1 tablespoon olive oil
- 1 small pinch salt and pepper
- ¼ cup low fat milk
- 8 eggs
- ½ teaspoon salt
- ¼ teaspoon pepper
- 3 ounces goat cheese or feta

Directions

1. Preheat the oven to 400°F.
2. Place the asparagus in a mixing bowl and drizzle with olive oil. Toss to coat then sprinkle with a pinch of salt and pepper. Arrange the asparagus in a single layer on foil-lined baking sheet
3. Roast until the asparagus is lightly charred and tender, about 10-15 minutes.
4. Take the asparagus out of the oven and set aside to cool slightly. (Leave oven at 400 degrees).

5. Cut into bite-sized pieces and set aside.
6. Using a fork, mix the eggs, milk, salt and pepper in a medium bowl and stir to combine. Set aside.
7. Pre-heat large non-stick, oven-safe pan over medium heat and add chopped asparagus to the pan. Cook the asparagus for 1 minute then add egg mixture into the pan.
8. Stir once with a rubber spatula then crumble goat cheese or feta over the top.
9. Last, transfer the pan to the preheated oven and bake 12-18 minutes or until eggs are set.
10. Remove from the oven and allow to cool slightly. Slice into 8 pieces and serve.
11. You can serve the frittata warm or cold. If you serve it cold, store it in an airtight container in the fridge.

Nutrition Facts

Per serving (1 slice) | Calories: 122 | Fat: 8g | Carbohydrates: 1.7g | Fiber: 0.6g | Sugars: 0.7g | Protein: 9.2g | Sodium: 250mg

Greek Yogurt Pumpkin Muffins

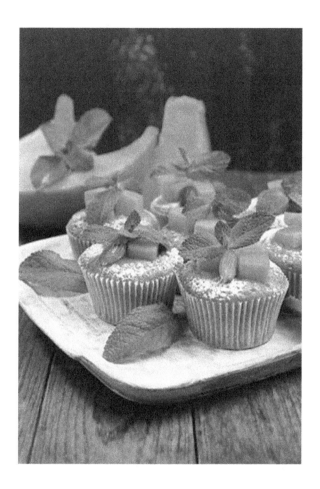

Preparation Time: 15 minutes

Cooking Time: 25-30 minutes

Yield: 16 muffins

Ingredients

- 2 eggs
- 2 cups pumpkin puree

- 2 cups nonfat plain Greek yogurt
- ¼ cup canola oil
- 1 teaspoon vanilla extract
- 2½ cups all-purpose flour
- 1½ cups sugar
- 1½ teaspoons cinnamon
- 1 teaspoon ground cloves
- 1 teaspoon baking soda
- ¼ teaspoon salt

Directions

1. Preheat oven to 350°F and grease 2 muffin tins with cooking spray.
2. Measure and place the flour, sugar, cinnamon, baking soda, cloves and salt in a large bowl and whisk together. Set aside.
3. In another bowl, whisk together the eggs, yogurt, pumpkin puree, oil and vanilla extract.
4. Add pumpkin mixture to the flour mixture and stir until combined. Do not overmix.
5. Scoop ¼ cup batter into each muffin well.
6. Bake until muffins spring back when pressed lightly on top and a toothpick inserted in the center of a muffin comes out clean, 25 to 30 minutes.
7. Cool 5 minutes in pan.

Nutrition Facts

Per serving (1 muffin) | Calories: 204 | Fat: 4g | Carbohydrates: 37g | Fiber: 1g | Sugars: 21g | Protein: 6g | Sodium: 132mg

Steel Cut Pumpkin-Apple-Spice Oatmeal

Preparation Time: 10 minutes

Cooking Time: 25-30 minutes

Yield: 4 servings

Ingredients

- 3 cups water
- 1 cup steel cut oats
- 1 cup pumpkin puree
- 1 teaspoon vanilla extract
- 1 teaspoon ground cinnamon
- ¼ teaspoon ground nutmeg
- ¼ teaspoon ground cloves
- 1 apple, peeled and grated

After cooking:

- 2 tablespoons maple syrup or more to sweeten
- 2 tablespoons pumpkin seeds/pepitas optional

Directions

1. Place steel cut oats, pumpkin puree, nutmeg, cloves, ground cinnamon, vanilla extract, and grated apple in a medium pot.

2. Add water, cover and bring to a boil then reduce to a simmer. Cook on low, stirring frequently, for 25-30 minutes, until cooked through.
3. Add maple syrup and stir to combine. Divide into bowls and top each with pumpkin seeds.

Nutrition Facts

Per serving (¼ of recipe) | Calories: 258 | Fat: 5g | Carbohydrates: 45g | Fiber: 7g | Sugars: 12g | Protein: 8g | Sodium: 15mg

Tropical Mango-Coconut Couscous Bowl

Preparation Time: 5 minutes

Cooking Time: 5 minutes

Yield: 4 servings

Ingredients

- 1 cup whole wheat couscous
- 1 cup 2% plain yogurt
- 2 cups milk
- ¼ cup chopped dried mango
- 2 tablespoons unsweetened shredded coconut (optional)
- 1 tablespoon packed brown sugar or liquid honey
- ½ teaspoon vanilla extract
- 2 bananas, sliced

Directions

1. Place mango, coconut (if using) and milk in a saucepan. Bring to almost a boil over medium heat, stirring often.
2. Add couscous and stir to combine. Cover tightly with a lid, remove from heat, and allow to sit for about 5 minutes.
3. Meanwhile, combine the yogurt, brown sugar (or honey), and vanilla in a bowl.
4. Fluff the couscous with a fork then add banana slices.

5. Divide into bowls and top with yogurt mixture.

Nutrition Facts

Per serving ($\frac{1}{4}$ of recipe) | Calories: 359 | Fat: 5g | Carbohydrates: 67g | Fiber: 6.3g | Protein: 14g | Sodium: 104mg

Creamy Avocado Mango Smoothie

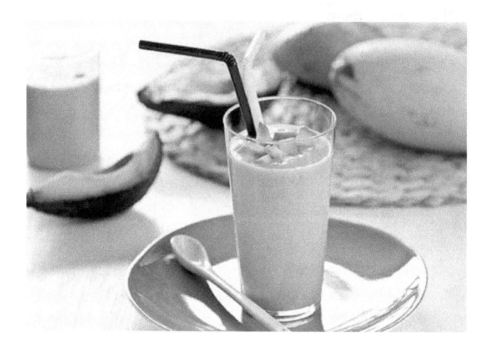

Preparation Time: 10 minutes

Cooking Time: 0 minutes

Yield: 2 servings

Ingredients

- ¼ ripe fresh avocado, seeded, peeled and diced
- ½ cup frozen mango cubes
- ⅓ cup plain, nonfat yogurt
- 1 tablespoon minced ginger
- 1 tablespoon lemon juice
- 1 cup water

- 1 cup ice cubes
- Cayenne pepper to taste (optional)

Directions

1. Place all the ingredients in the blender and blend until smooth.
2. Serve and enjoy!

Nutrition Facts

Per serving (½ of recipe) | Calories: 90 | Fat: 3.5g | Carbohydrates: 13g | Fiber: 2g | Sugars: 9g | Protein: 5g | Sodium: 25mg

Healthy Egg Muffin Cups

Preparation Time: 15 minutes

Cooking Time: 25 minutes

Yield: 12 muffins

Ingredients

- 1 cup lightly packed baby spinach, chopped
- ¾ cup finely diced green bell pepper(about 1 small pepper)
- ¾ cup finely diced red bell pepper(about 1 small pepper)
- ¾ cup quartered cherry tomatoes or grape tomatoes (about 1 cup whole tomatoes)
- 6 large eggs
- 4 large egg whites
- ¼ teaspoon dried basil
- ¼ teaspoon dried oregano
- ¼ teaspoon kosher salt
- Pinch ground black pepper
- ¼ cup crumbled feta cheese, plus additional to sprinkle on top

Directions

1. Place a rack in the center of your oven and preheat to 350°F. Spray a 12-cup muffin tin with nonstick cooking spray.
2. Divide the green bell pepper, red bell pepper, spinach, and tomatoes among the cups.
3. Ina large mixing bowl, combine eggs, egg whites, salt, basil, oregano, and pepper and whisk well.
4. Fill each muffin cup ¾ full with the egg mixture, pouring over the vegetables.
5. Sprinkle Feta over the top of each muffin.
6. Bake for 24 to 28 minutes, until the egg muffins are set.
7. Once cooked, let them cool for 5-7 minutes then run a small butter knife around the edges of each muffin to loosen. Remove from pan and serve!

Nutrition Facts

Per serving (1 muffin) | Calories: 70 | Fat: 3g | Carbohydrates: 3g | Fiber: 1g | Sugars: 2g | Protein: 8g | Sodium: 148mg

Easy Banana Chocolate Chip Muffins

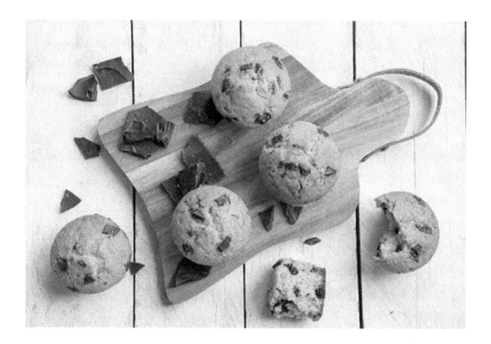

Preparation Time: 15 minutes

Cooking Time: 20 minutes

Yield: 15 muffins

Ingredients

- 2 cups white whole wheat flour
- 1 teaspoon salt
- ½ teaspoon baking powder
- ½ teaspoon ground cinnamon
- ½ teaspoon baking soda
- ½ teaspoon ground nutmeg

- 2 large eggs
- ⅔ cup vegetable oil
- ¼ cup stevia
- 1 tablespoon vanilla extract
- 3 ripe bananas, mashed
- ¾ cup mini chocolate chips, divided

Directions

1. Preheat oven to 350°F.
2. Linea12-cup muffin tin with paper muffin cases.
3. Put the flour, baking powder, baking soda, salt, nutmeg and cinnamon in a large bowl. Mix them.
4. In another bowl, put the stevia, eggs, oil and vanilla and whisk them. Fold in bananas until combined.
5. Pour the wet ingredients into the dry and mix with a wooden spoon or rubber spatula until combined. Stir in ½ cup chocolate chips.
6. Spoon the batter evenly into the muffin pan, filling each cup about ¾ full. Sprinkle with remaining ¼ cup chocolate chips.
7. Bake at 350°F for 15-17 minutes or until a toothpick inserted in the center comes out clean.
8. Remove from oven and cool on a wire rack.

Nutrition Facts

Per serving (1 muffin) | Calories: 203 | Fat: 12g | Carbohydrates: 23g | Fiber: 0g | Sugars: 8g | Protein: 2g | Sodium: 122mg

Chocolate Raspberry Overnight Oats

Preparation Time: 20 minutes + Soak Time (overnight)

Cooking Time: 10 minutes

Yield: 4 servings

Ingredients

For the Raspberry Chia Seed Jam (makes 1 cup):

- 1 (10 oz.) bag frozen raspberries
- 2 tablespoons chia seeds
- 2 tablespoons pure maple syrup, or to taste
- 1 teaspoon pure vanilla extract or vanilla bean powder (optional)

For the Chocolate Overnight Oats (makes 3 cups):

- 1 cup gluten-free rolled oats
- 2½ cups unsweetened almond milk
- ⅓ cup chia seeds
- 2 to 3 tablespoons pure maple syrup, to taste
- 2 tablespoons unsweetened cocoa powder

For the topping*:

- Fresh or frozen raspberries
- Sliced toasted almonds or hazelnuts

Directions

1. *For the Raspberry Chia Seed Jam:* Combine the raspberries, chia seeds, and maple syrup in a medium-sized pot. Stir to combine. Cook uncovered over medium heat, stirring frequently, about 7 to 9 minutes, until the berries break down.
Remove from heat and add the vanilla, if using. Set aside, uncovered, about 30 minutes to cool completely. Cover and transfer to the fridge.
2. *For the Chocolate Overnight Oats*: In a bowl, stir together cocoa powder and 3-4 tablespoons of the milk until combined and there are no chunks of cocoa powder. Add remaining milk, chia seeds, and maple syrup. Mix. Add the rolled oats and mix again. Close the lid and set aside for 2-3 minutes. Then stir again, cover and put the container in the fridge overnight.
3. When the chia jam and oats are ready, layer them in jars or bowls. Add your desired toppings, and enjoy!

*Nutrition Information does not include toppings, such as nuts and fresh/frozen berries.

Nutrition Facts

Per serving (¼ of recipe) | Calories: 320 | Fat: 11g | Carbohydrates: 50g | Fiber: 16g | Sugars: 16g | Protein: 9g | Sodium: 180mg

Crustless Broccoli Cheddar Quiche

Preparation Time: 10 minutes

Cooking Time: 40-45 minutes

Yield: 8 slices

Ingredients

- 3 cups broccoli florets, chopped (about 1 large head)
- 1 cup grated cheddar
- 6 eggs
- 1 cup milk or cream
- 1 teaspoon garlic, minced
- ½ teaspoon salt
- ¼ teaspoon cayenne

Directions

1. Preheat oven to 350°F.
2. Butter a 9-inch pie plate and set aside.
3. Prepare the egg filling: In a mixing bowl, combine the eggs, milk, garlic, salt and cayenne and whisk until combined. Add cheese and stir.
4. Evenly spread the broccoli in the dish and pour the egg mixture on top.
5. Place in the middle of the preheated oven. Bake uncovered for 40-45 minutes or until firm and golden.
6. Let cool for about 10 minutes then slice into wedges and serve.

Nutrition Facts

Per serving (1 slice) | Calories: 160 | Fat: 10g | Carbohydrates: 7g | Fiber: 2g | Sugars: 1g | Protein: 11g | Sodium: 319mg

Dinner Recipes

Stuffed Portobello Mushrooms

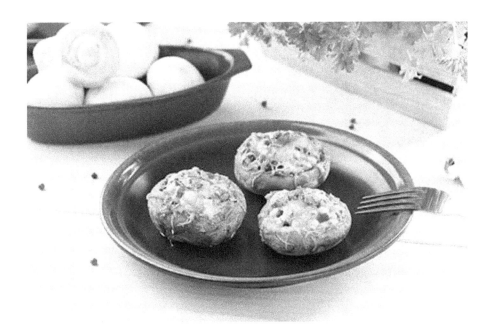

Preparation Time: 15 minutes

Cooking Time: 30 minutes

Yield: 4 servings

Ingredients

- 4 medium-sized portobello mushrooms
- 1 tablespoon olive oil, divided
- ½ red onion, diced
- 2 chicken breasts (or 2 cups leftover cooked chicken)

- ½ red pepper, diced
- 1 egg
- ¼ cup breadcrumbs
- 2 cloves garlic, minced
- ¼ cup fresh parsley, chopped, plus more for garnish
- 1 cup shredded cheddar cheese, divided
- ½ teaspoon each salt & pepper

Directions

1. Preheat oven to 400°F.
2. Toss chicken breasts with ½ tablespoon olive oil, ¼ teaspoon salt each and pepper. Mix well to coat. Place on a lightly greased pan and bake 15-18 minutes until chicken is barely cooked through. Let cool then shred or chop into small pieces.
3. Change oven temperature to 350°F.
4. De-stem and scrape out the portobellos, reserving inside mushroom gills and disposing of stems.
5. Place mushroom gills in a large bowl and add cooked chicken, red pepper, red onion, egg, breadcrumbs, parsley, garlic and half the cheese. Season with ¼ teaspoon salt and pepper and toss to combine.
6. Divide filling among mushroom caps. Sprinkle with remaining cheese.
7. Arrange the mushrooms on a baking sheet and bake in oven for 18-20 minutes until mushroom caps are cooked through and cheese is melted.

8. Garnish with a sprinkle of parsley.
9. Serve and enjoy!

Nutrition Facts

Per serving (1 mushroom) | Calories: 313 | Fat: 14g | Carbohydrates: 10g | Fiber: 1g | Sugars: 3g | Protein: 35g | Sodium: 380mg

Simple Turkey Salad with Arugula and Grapes

Preparation Time: 20 minutes

Cooking Time: 0 minutes

Yield: 6 servings

Ingredients

For the Dressing:

- ½ cup orange juice
- 3 tablespoons red wine vinegar
- 3 tablespoons sesame oil
- 2 tablespoons minced fresh chives
- ¼ teaspoon salt
- ¼ teaspoon ground black pepper

For the Salad:

- 4 cups cooked turkey, cubed
- 4 teaspoons curry powder
- ¼ teaspoon salt
- ½ teaspoon freshly ground pepper
- 3 cups fresh arugula or baby spinach
- 1 large apple, chopped
- 1 cup green grapes, halved
- 1 can (11 ounces) mandarin oranges, drained

- ½ cup chopped walnuts
- ½ cup pomegranate seeds

Directions

1. To make the dressing, combine the orange juice, sesame oil, minced chives and red wine vinegar in a bowl. Sprinkle with salt and pepper. Mix to combine.
2. In a separate large bowl, combine the cubed turkey with curry powder, salt and pepper. Toss to coat. Add grapes, apple, arugula and mandarin oranges.
3. Drizzle dressing over salad and gently toss to coat evenly. Scatter walnuts and pomegranate seeds on top.
4. Serve immediately.

Nutrition Facts

Per serving | Calories: 354 | Fat: 17g| Carbohydrates: 22g | Fiber: 3g | Sugars: 17g | Protein: 30g | Sodium: 301 mg

Roasted Sweet Potato & Avocado Salad

Preparation Time: 5 minutes

Cooking Time: 25 minutes

Yield: 1 serving

Ingredients

For the Sweet Potato:

- 1 large (or 2 small) organic sweet potatoes (skin on, halved then sliced into ¼-inch rounds)
- 1 tablespoon avocado or coconut oil
- 1 pinch sea salt

For the Dressing:

- ¼ cup tahini (sesame seed paste)
- 2 tablespoons lemon juice
- 1 tablespoon maple syrup (optional)
- 1 pinch sea salt
- Water (to thin)

For the Salad:

- 5 cups greens of choice (I mixed arugula + spinach)
- 1 medium ripe avocado (cubed)
- 2 tablespoons hemp seeds

Directions

1. Preheat oven to 375°F.
2. Place sweet potato slices in a large bowl, sprinkle with salt, and toss. In the same bowl, drizzle oil over the sweet potato slices and toss again until they are evenly coated. Arrange in a single layer on a baking sheet lined with parchment paper.
3. Bake 15 minutes then flip them and bake an additional 5-10minutes or until tender and golden brown.
4. Meanwhile, in a small bowl, combine lemon juice, tahini, maple syrup, and salt; stir until well-blended. Then add water a little at a time until a semi-thick, pourable dressing is achieved.
5. Adjust if necessary – if you'd like more tang, add more lemon, or for more overall flavor, add another pinch of salt. Set aside.
6. Place greens, avocado and sweet potatoes in a serving bowl. Pour the dressing over the salad and sprinkle with hemp seeds. Enjoy!

Nutrition Facts

Per serving | Calories: 663 | Fat: 45.6g | Carbohydrates: 49.8g | Fiber: 17.9g | Sugars: 12.9g | Protein: 22.3g | Sodium: 275mg

Quinoa Stuffed Bell Peppers

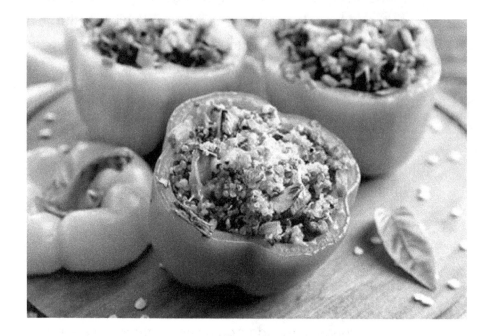

Preparation Time: 15 minutes

Cooking Time: 1 hour 40 minutes

Yield: 4 servings

Ingredients

- 4 bell peppers (any color)
- 3 tablespoons extra virgin olive oil
- 1 yellow onion, chopped
- 1 clove garlic, chopped
- ½ teaspoon kosher salt
- 1 pint grape tomatoes, cut in half
- 2 cups coarsely chopped collard greens

- 1 cup quinoa
- ¼ teaspoon crushed red pepper flakes
- 1 cup fresh corn kernels
- ¼ teaspoon freshly ground black pepper

Directions

1. Heat the oven to 375°F.
2. Place a large saucepan over medium heat and add 2 tablespoons of olive oil. Once the oil is heated, add garlic and onion then sprinkle with ¼ teaspoon of salt. Cover with lid and cook, stirring often, 5 to 6 minutes or until tender.
3. Add tomatoes, cover again, and cook stirring occasionally, about 8 minutes or until the tomatoes have softened.
4. Stir in the collard greens and cook, covered, for 2 minutes to soften.
5. Add the quinoa into the tomato mixture. Pour in 2 cups of water; add red pepper flakes and the remaining ¼ teaspoon salt; bring to a boil.
6. Cover with lid, turn the heat down to low, and simmer for 12 to 15 minutes or until the quinoa is tender and liquid has been soaked in completely.
7. Turn off heat and let stand, covered, 5 to 7 minutes.
8. Stir in the corn and sprinkle with black pepper.
9. Cut each pepper around the stem just below the "shoulders" and remove to create a lid. Remove and

discard membranes and seeds and, if the peppers do not sit flat, trim the bottoms slightly.

10. Generously stuff peppers with quinoa-vegetable mixture until all peppers are full. Place the stuffed peppers in a baking dish and cover with their reserved tops. Drizzle 1 tablespoon of olive oil over the pepper cups and lids.

11. Add 1½ cups of water into the dish. Bake in the preheated oven until bell peppers are tender, about 1 hour.

12. Serve hot or room temperature.

Nutrition Facts

Per serving | Calories: 276 | Fat: 13g | Carbohydrates: 34g | Fiber: 6g | Sugars: 8g | Protein: 7g | Sodium: 280mg

Pan Seared Fish with Creamy Spinach

Preparation Time: 5 minutes

Cooking Time: 15 minutes

Yield: 4 servings

Ingredients

- 4 (5 oz. thick) pieces of white firm fish fillet (bass or halibut),skinless
- 1 tablespoon extra virgin olive oil
- 1 tablespoon unsalted butter
- 1 cup red bell pepper, chopped
- 2 cloves garlic, minced
- 9 ounces fresh baby spinach
- ¼ cup half & half cream
- 2 ounces ⅓ less fat cream cheese
- 3 tablespoons Parmesan cheese, grated
- fresh black pepper, to taste
- kosher salt, to taste

Directions

1. Place a large skillet over medium heat and add ½ tablespoon of olive oil and ½ tablespoon of butter. Stir in chopped red bell pepper and garlic. Cook, stirring occasionally, about 4 minutes.

2. Add spinach, sprinkle with a little pinch of salt and pepper, and cook, tossing often, until spinach is wilted, 2 to 3 minutes.
3. Stir in half & half, cream cheese and parmesan cheese. Mix well until cream cheese is melted and smooth.
4. Place a separate skillet over medium-high heat and add the remaining olive oil and butter.
5. Sprinkle both sides of fish with a little pinch of salt and pepper and add to the hot pan. Fry until bottom is golden, 6 minutes, then flip it over to cook for anadditional5 minutes until cooked through and browned.
6. Transfer the spinach to individual plates and top with the fish.

Nutrition Facts

Per serving | Calories: 351 | Fat: 16.5g | Carbohydrates: 6g | Fiber: 2g | Sugars: 2g | Protein: 43g | Sodium: 300mg

Tuna Corn Salad

Preparation Time: 15 minutes + chilling time (15-20 minutes)

Cooking Time: 15 minutes

Yield: 4 servings

Ingredients

- 1 teaspoon olive oil
- ½ cup nonfat Greek yogurt
- 1 large ear corn
- ½ teaspoon oregano
- 1 teaspoon chili powder
- ½ teaspoon ground cumin
- ¼ teaspoon salt
- ½ lime (juiced)
- 1 small red bell pepper (seeded and diced)
- 1 small jalapeno (finely minced)
- 2 medium ribs celery (diced)
- 1 (15 oz.) can no salt added black beans (drained and rinsed)
- 2 (5 oz.) cans no salt added tuna (drained)

Directions

1. Slice the kernels from the cob with a sharp knife.
2. In a large skillet, heat olive oil over medium high heat.

3. Add corn; cook 12 to 15 minutes or until corn starts to brown, stirring occasionally.
4. Once the corn is browned, transfer it to a small bowl then refrigerate 15 to 20 minutes while you prepare the sauce.
5. Stir together yogurt, cumin, chili powder, oregano, lime juice, and salt in a bowl until smooth. Let it chill in the fridge for 10-15 minutes.
6. When the corn and the sauce have chilled, place them together in a large mixing bowl. Add black beans, celery, jalapeno, red pepper, and tuna.
7. Lightly toss the ingredients until coated and serve.

Nutrition Facts

Per serving (about 1½ cups) | Calories: 269 | Fat: 4g | Carbohydrates: 29g | Fiber: 9g | Sugars: 4g | Protein: 29g | Sodium: 233mg

Sirloin Steak with Roasted Potatoes and Broccoli

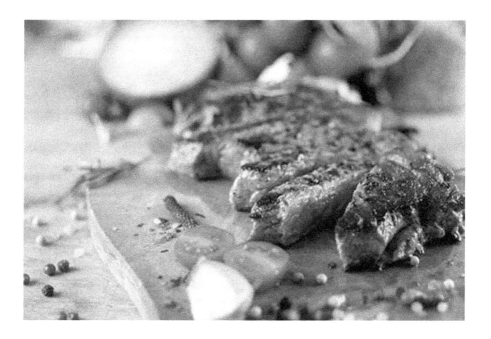

Preparation Time: 15 minutes

Cooking Time: 15 minutes

Yield: 6 servings

Ingredients

- 2 pounds baby red potatoes
- 16 ounces broccoli florets (about 3 cups)
- 2 pounds (1-inch-thick) top sirloin steak, patted dry
- 3 cloves garlic, minced
- 1 teaspoon dried thyme
- 2 tablespoons olive oil

- Kosher salt and freshly ground black pepper, to taste

Directions

1. Preheat oven to broil. Grease a baking sheet with oil.
2. Add potatoes to a large pot then pour over enough water to cover potatoes by 1 inch. Season with a teaspoon of salt per pound of potatoes. Bring water to a boil over high heat; boil the potatoes for about 12-15 minutes then drain.
3. Add the potatoes to a large mixing bowl and drizzle with olive oil. Add the minced garlic, thyme, broccoli, salt, and pepper. Mix well to combine.
4. Season steaks with salt and pepper to taste.
5. Spread the potato mixture and steaks in a single layer on the baking sheet.
6. Place into oven and broil about 5-6 minutes. Then flip steaks and broil another 5-6 minutes until the steak is browned and charred at the edges.
7. Remove from oven and place on a serving plate.

Nutrition Facts

Per serving (⅙ of recipe) | Calories: 460.3 | Fat: 24g | Carbohydrates: 24g | Fiber: 2.6g | Sugars: 1.3g | Protein: 36g | Sodium: 108mg

Zucchini Pasta with Avocado Sauce

Preparation Time: 15 minutes

Cooking Time: 5 minutes

Yield: 2 servings

Ingredients

For the sauce:

- 1 ripe avocado
- 1 lime, juiced
- 2 tablespoons cilantro, chopped
- 1 teaspoon jalapeno, minced
- 1 small clove of garlic, minced
- Pinch of salt and pepper
- Water to thin, if needed

For the rest:

- 2 medium zucchinis
- 2 teaspoons olive oil
- 1 medium ear of corn, kernels shaved off
- ½ teaspoon chili powder
- 1 cup cherry tomatoes, halved
- Pinch of salt and pepper

Directions

1. Place a medium skillet over medium-high heat and add olive oil. Once the oil is heated, add the corn and season with salt, pepper, and chili powder. Cook until corn is cooked through and fork tender, about 5 minutes. Set aside when done.
2. Cut avocado in half, remove the pit, and peel off the skin. Add avocado and remaining sauce ingredients to the bowl of a food processor. Pulse until mixture is smooth and creamy.
3. Trim the ends of the zucchini. Use a vegetable peeler or spiralizer to make long, thin strips of zucchini.
4. Put the zucchini noodles with the sauce into a bowl and toss to coat.
5. Place the coated zucchini on serving plates and top with corn and tomatoes.

Nutrition Facts

Per serving (½ of recipe) | Calories: 329 | Fat: 25g | Carbohydrates: 37g | Fiber: 15g | Sugars: 12g | Protein: 9g | Sodium: 232mg

Beet & Orange Salad

Preparation Time: 15 minutes

Cooking Time: 1 hour + cooling

Yield: 4 servings

Ingredients

- 2 medium fresh beets
- 1 package (5 ounces) mixed salad greens
- 1 small fennel bulb, halved and thinly sliced
- $\frac{1}{4}$ cup chopped hazelnuts, toasted
- 2 medium navel oranges, peeled and sliced

Dressing:

- 3 tablespoons olive oil
- 1 tablespoon balsamic vinegar
- $\frac{1}{4}$ teaspoon onion powder
- 2 teaspoons grated orange zest
- 2 tablespoons orange juice

Directions

1. Preheat oven to 425°F.
2. Trim the ends of the beets. Place on a baking sheet, cut a few slits in beets, and bake in oven for an hour or until beets are pierced easily with a paring knife.

3. When the beets are cooked, remove them from the oven and allow them to cool until they're safe to handle. Once the beets are cool enough to handle, peel them and cut into slices or wedges (you can wear disposable gloves to handle the beets if you don't want beet-stained fingers).
4. Divide greens among serving plates; top with oranges, beets, fennel and hazelnuts.
5. In the mason jar, add all the dressing ingredients. Screw on the lid and shake the jar until fully combined.
6. Pour dressing over salad.

Nutrition Facts

Per serving (¼ of recipe) | Calories: 213 | Fat: 15g | Carbohydrates: 21g | Fiber: 6g | Sugars: 12g | Protein: 4g | Sodium: 80mg

Creamy Mashed Potatoes

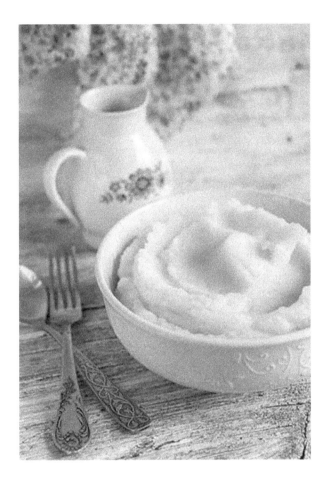

Preparation Time: 15 minutes

Cooking Time: 1 hour

Yield: 6 servings

Ingredients

- 4 to 5 large potatoes (about 2-$\frac{1}{2}$pounds)

- ½ cup sour cream
- 3 ounces cream cheese, softened
- 1 tablespoon chopped chives
- ¼ teaspoon black pepper
- 1 tablespoon butter
- ¾ teaspoon onion salt
- Paprika, optional

Directions

1. Peel the potatoes, removing all dark spots. Cut the potatoes into cubes then add to a large saucepan and cover with cold water by an inch.
2. Bring to a boil over medium heat, cover loosely, and cook approximately15 to 20 minutes or until potatoes break apart easily when pierced with a fork.
3. Drain the potatoes then return them to the pan. Use a potato masher to mash potatoes until smooth.
4. Add cream cheese, sour cream, chives, onion salt and pepper; beat until fluffy.
5. Transfer to a greased 1-½-quart baking dish. Dot with butter and sprinkle with paprika.
6. Cover and bake at 350°F for 35-40 minutes or until heated through.

Nutrition Facts

Per serving (¾ cup) | Calories: 301 | Fat: 10g |
Carbohydrates: 45g | Fiber: 4g |Sugars: 5g | Protein: 7g |
Sodium: 313mg

Zucchini Casserole

Preparation Time: 15 minutes

Cooking Time: 30 minutes

Yield: 6 servings

Ingredients

- 2 medium zucchini and/or summer squash, sliced
- 2 medium tomatoes, sliced
- ¼ cup chopped basil plus 2 tablespoons, divided
- 1 tablespoon extra-virgin olive oil
- ¼ cup finely chopped shallot
- ¾ cup shredded fresh mozzarella cheese (3 ounces)
- ½ teaspoon salt
- ¼ teaspoon ground pepper

Directions

1. Preheat oven to 400°F.
2. Spray 8x8-inchbaking dish with cooking spray.
3. Places quash and tomato slices in baking dish, creating overlapping rows.
4. Combine shallot, oil, ¼ cup basil, salt and pepper in a small bowl. Pour the mixture over the vegetables.

5. Top with shredded mozzarella cheese and bake about 30 minutes or until the vegetables are tender and the cheese has melted.
6. Remove from the oven and strew remaining chopped basil over the top.

Nutrition Facts

Per serving (¾ cup) | Calories: 87 | Fat: 5g | Carbohydrates: 6g | Fiber: 1g | Sugars: 3g | Protein: 5g | Sodium: 296mg

Farro Salad with Chickpeas and Feta

Preparation Time: 5 minutes

Cooking Time: 0 minutes

Yield: 1 serving

Ingredients

Dressing:

- 2 teaspoons extra-virgin olive oil
- 2 teaspoons red wine vinegar
- ½ small garlic clove, grated
- ⅛ teaspoon dried oregano

Salad:

- 1 cup arugula
- ¼ cup diced red bell pepper
- ½ cup cooked unpearled farro
- ¼ cup diced cucumber
- ⅓ cup canned unsalted chickpeas, rinsed and drained
- 2 tablespoons feta cheese, crumbled

Directions

1. Combine all salad ingredients in a large mixing bowl.

2. Then place all the dressing ingredients in a small bowl and whisk to combine; drizzle over salad and toss to coat.
3. To serve, place the salad in a serving bowl.

Nutrition Facts

Per serving | Calories: 341 | Fat: 15g | Carbohydrates: 46g | Fiber: 8g | Sugars: 4g | Protein: 12.5g | Sodium: 238mg

Vegetable Salad with Lime Dressing

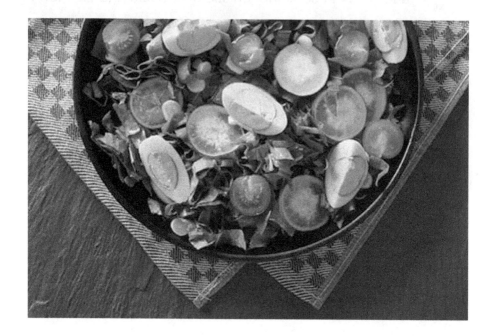

Preparation Time: 10 minutes

Yield: 6 servings

Ingredients

- 3 tablespoons lime juice
- ¼ cup canola oil
- ¼ cup extra-virgin olive oil
- 1½ tablespoons fresh cilantro, finely chopped
- ½ teaspoon ground pepper
- ½ teaspoon salt
- 6 leaves romaine or leaf lettuce

- 2 cups mixed vegetables (Steamed: sliced small red potatoes, carrots or beets, green beans, peas; Raw: sliced radishes, cucumbers or tomatoes)
- 1 small bunch watercress, large stems removed
- 1 hard-boiled large egg, sliced
- 1 thick slice red onion, broken into rings
- Crumbled Mexican queso fresco, feta or farmer's cheese for garnish

Directions

1. To make the dressing, combine lime juice, canola oil, olive oil, cilantro, salt and pepper in a medium bowl. Mix to combine.
2. Stir in mixed vegetables and toss to coat.
3. Arrange lettuce leaves on a serving platter or individual plates.
4. Spoon the dressed vegetables over lettuce, garnish with watercress, and top with egg, onion and cheese, if desired.

Nutrition Facts

Per serving (1½ cups) | Calories: 214 | Fat: 20g | Carbohydrates: 8g | Fiber: 2g | Sugars: 2g | Protein: 3g | Sodium: 217mg

Greek Orzo Salad

Preparation Time: 15 minutes

Yield: 6 servings

Ingredients

- 8 ounces dried orzo pasta, cooked in salted water according to package directions, then cooled
- 1½ cups cucumber, diced
- 1 cup cherry tomatoes, halved
- 1 cup chickpeas, rinsed and drained
- ½ cup feta cheese, crumbled
- ¼ cup chopped fresh parsley
- ¼ cup minced red onion

Dressing:

- 6 tablespoons olive oil
- 1 tablespoon red wine vinegar
- 1 tablespoon lemon juice
- 1 teaspoon Dijon mustard
- ¼ teaspoon garlic powder
- ¼ teaspoon dried oregano
- Pinch of salt and pepper

Directions

1. Combine the orzo pasta, chickpeas, cucumber, parsley, cherry tomatoes, red onion and feta cheese in a large mixing bowl.
2. Then place all the dressing ingredients in a small bowl and whisk to combine; pour over pasta mixture and toss to coat.
3. To serve, place the orzo salad in serving bowls.

Nutrition Facts

Per serving (⅙ of recipe) | Calories: 310 | Fat: 13g | Carbohydrates: 38g | Fiber: 3g | Sugars: 4g | Protein: 9g | Sodium: 157mg

Mushroom Cauliflower Rice Casserole

Preparation Time: 20 minutes

Cooking Time: 40-45 minutes

Yield: 8 servings

Ingredients

- 16 oz. cremini mushrooms, sliced
- 16 oz. riced cauliflower(fresh, not frozen)
- 2 cups Brussels sprouts, quartered(about8 oz.)
- 1 medium apple, cored and diced
- 2 medium carrots, chopped
- 2 celery ribs, sliced
- 1 small yellow onion, chopped
- 3 cloves garlic, minced
- 3 tablespoons olive or avocado oil
- 1½ teaspoons fresh thyme(or ½ teaspoon dried)
- 1½ teaspoons fresh rosemary, minced(or 1 teaspoon dried, lightly chopped or crushed)
- 1½ tablespoons fresh sage, minced (or ¾ teaspoon dried)
- ¾ teaspoon salt
- ⅓ cup pecans, chopped and toasted
- ½ cup no-sugar-added dried cranberries
- Black pepper, to taste

Directions

1. Preheat oven to 375°F.
2. Spray with nonstick cooking spray or lightly grease bottom of 9x13-inch baking dish.
3. Place all the ingredients (except dried fruit and pecans) in prepared baking dish and toss gently until combined.
4. Cover dish with aluminum foil and bake in the preheated oven for 30 minutes.
5. Uncover; stir and bake uncovered an additional 10-15 minutes until vegetables are tender.
6. Add dried fruit and toasted pecans just before serving.

Nutrition Facts

Per serving (1 cup) | Calories: 137 | Fat: 9g | Carbohydrates: 13g | Fiber: 4g | Sugars: 6g | Protein: 4g | Sodium: 262mg

Tuna Salad Avocado Boats

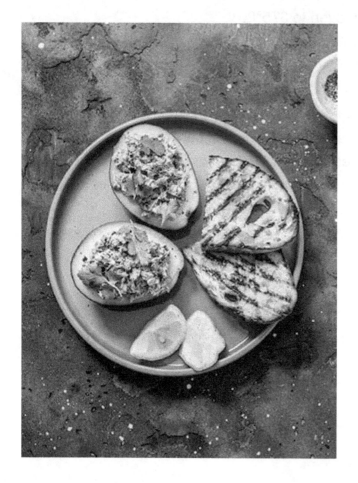

Preparation Time: 5 minutes

Yield: 2 servings

Ingredients

- 1 avocado
- 5 ounces cooked or canned tuna (low sodium)
- 1 lemon, juiced

- 1 tablespoon chopped sweet onion
- Fresh ground black pepper, to taste
- Pinch of sea salt

Directions

1. Slice the avocado in half and remove the pit. Scoop half of the flesh out of each avocado half (leave half undisturbed) and transfer to a bowl.
2. Add lemon juice and onion to the avocado in the bowl and mash with a fork. Stir in tuna. Season with salt and pepper and stir to combine. Taste and adjust if needed.
3. Spoon the tuna mixture equally into each avocado half.
4. Serve

Nutrition Facts

Per serving ($\frac{1}{2}$ of recipe) | Calories: 239 | Fat: 15g | Carbohydrates: 14g | Fiber: 8g | Sugars: 2g | Protein: 16g | Sodium: 183mg

Broccoli Salad with Creamy Cashew Dressing

Preparation Time: 15 minutes + soaking time if needed

Cooking Time: 15 minutes

Yield: 6 servings

Ingredients

Creamy Cashew Sauce:

- 1 cup raw cashews
- 1 cup unsweetened coconut milk (from a carton)
- 2 tablespoons maple syrup(or agave)
- 2 tablespoons apple cider vinegar
- 1 tablespoon lemon juice (about ½ a large lemon)
- ⅛ teaspoon black pepper (more to taste)
- ¼ teaspoon sea salt

Broccoli Salad:

- 2 lbs. raw broccoli, florets cut into small bite sized pieces*
- ½ cup red onion, diced
- ¼ cup roasted pumpkin seeds
- ½ cup dried cherries
- 1 cup grapes, halved

Directions

1. You can choose to boil or soak the cashews.
   To soak the cashews: Place the raw cashews in a bowl. Cover with cold filtered water and soak for about 2hours.
   To boil the cashews: Place the raw cashews in a medium saucepan and cover with water. Bring to a boil over high heat then reduce the heat to medium; cook10-15minutes, until the cashews are very tender.
2. Drain the cashews and discard the water.
3. Place the soaked cashews, lemon juice, coconut milk, apple cider vinegar, maple syrup, salt, and pepper into the bowl of a food processor. Blend until smooth and creamy.
4. Place the broccoli, cherries, grapes, red onion and pumpkin seeds in a bowl.
5. Pour the cashew dressing over the salad and toss to coat.
6. Refrigerate the broccoli salad for one hour before serving.
7. Enjoy!

*Note: This salad is the perfect way to eat raw broccoli, but If you prefer broccoli to be softer, feel free to blanch it first.

Nutrition Facts

Per serving (⅙ of recipe) | Calories: 365 | Fat: 22g | Carbohydrates: 37g | Fiber: 7g | Sugars: 19g | Protein: 12g | Sodium: 171mg

Lunch Recipes

Couscous with Zucchini and Tomatoes

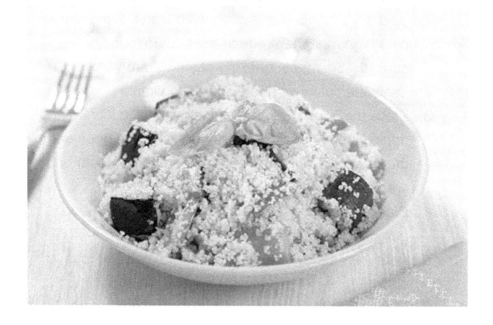

Preparation Time: 15 minutes

Cooking Time: 15 minutes

Yield: 6 servings

Ingredients

- 1½ teaspoons olive oil
- 1 large onion
- 1 large garlic clove, minced
- 2½ cups canned low-salt chicken broth

- 1½ pounds medium zucchini, trimmed, each cut crosswise into 3 pieces, each piece cut into 6 wedges
- 3 tablespoons chopped fresh thyme or 1 tablespoon dried
- 1½ cups couscous
- 1½ teaspoons butter
- 24 cherry tomatoes

Directions

1. Place a large saucepan over medium heat and add olive oil. Once the oil is heated, add onion and garlic. Cook, stirring often, 4-5 minutes or until tender and golden. Pour in broth and bring to boil.
2. Add zucchini and cook about 3 minutes or until the zucchini is crisp-tender.
3. Add couscous, thyme and butter; stir to combine, cover with a lid or a plate, and remove from the heat. Set aside for 5-7 minutes, until broth is absorbed. Then remove the lid and fluff with a fork.
4. Stir in tomatoes. If desired, garnish with thyme sprigs. Serve warm.

Nutrition Facts

Per serving (⅙ of recipe) | Calories: 242 | Fat: 4g | Carbohydrates: 44g | Fiber: 5g | Sugars: 2g | Protein: 10g | Sodium: 48mg

Grilled Tuna Mango Kabobs

Preparation Time: 15 minutes + Soak Time (10-15 minutes)

Cooking Time: 10-12 minutes

Yield: 4 servings

Ingredients

For the Salsa:

- ½ cup frozen corn, thawed
- 2 tablespoons coarsely chopped fresh parsley
- 4 green onions, chopped
- 1 jalapeno pepper, seeded and chopped
- 2 tablespoons lime juice

For the Kabobs:

- 1 pound tuna steaks, cut into 1-inch cubes
- 1 teaspoon coarsely ground pepper
- 2 large sweet red peppers, cut into 2x1-inch pieces
- 1 medium mango, peeled and cut into 1-inch cubes

Directions

1. Soak four 12-inch wooden skewers for at least 10 minutes in cold water to keep them from charring or use metal skewers.

2. To make the salsa: In a small bowl, combine corn, onions, parsley and jalapeño. Add lime juice and stir gently to combine. Set aside.
3. Rub tuna with pepper.
4. Thread tuna alternating with mango and red pepper on metal or soaked wooden skewer*.
5. Lightly spray the grill rack with cooking spray. Place skewers on grill rack. Grill, covered, over medium heat, turning occasionally, until tuna is slightly pink in the center (medium-rare) and peppers are tender, 10-12 minutes.
6. Transfer skewers to a serving plate and serve with salsa.

*Note: Select pieces of mango & red peppers that are close to the same size as your fish. This is important because, if the pieces are different widths, some things will be charred and others under cooked. Don't crowd the skewer, or the parts that are touching will cook too slowly.

Nutrition Facts

Per serving (1 kabob) | Calories: 205 | Fat: 2g | Carbohydrates: 20g | Fiber: 4g | Sugars: 12g | Protein: 29g | Sodium: 50mg

Sweet Potato Pasta with Avocado Sauce

Preparation Time: 15 minutes

Cooking Time: 10 minutes

Yield: 4 servings

Ingredients

- 3 medium sized sweet potatoes, peeled and spiralized
- 1 tablespoon extra virgin olive oil
- 1 clove garlic, crushed
- 1 (15 oz.) can chickpeas, drained and rinsed
- 1 tablespoon fresh basil, chopped
- 1 tablespoon lemon juice + zest from half lemon
- 1 teaspoon dried oregano
- ¼ cup pepitas/hulled pumpkin seeds
- crumbled up feta (dairy free/vegan if needed)

For the Avocado Tahini Sauce:

- 1 medium ripe avocado
- ¼ cup tahini
- 1 small handful basil (don't worry about being exact)
- 1 tablespoon lemon juice
- 2-3 tablespoons water (+ more as needed)

Directions

1. Peel the sweet potatoes. Slice in half and cut off the pointy tips. Place in the spiralizer and spiralize into noodles. Alternatively, you can use a julienne peeler to cut the sweet potatoes in very thin strips.
2. To make the sauce, place avocado, tahini, lemon juice and basil into a food processor. Pulse, then add water and blend until creamy. Set aside.
3. Place a large skillet over medium-low heat and add olive oil. Once the oil is heated, add garlic and sauté for a minute until fragrant, stirring constantly.
4. Add the sweet potato noodles and chickpeas. Cook, stirring frequently, 2-3 minutes or until noodles start to soften and are tender but still have a crisp "al dente" bite.
5. Add the lemon juice, zest, basil, oregano and pepitas and cook an additional 2 minutes. Remove from heat.
6. Add about half of the avocado tahini sauce to the noodles and toss to coat.*
7. To serve, divide noodles between plates. Top with feta and enjoy!

*Note: Store the remaining sauce in an airtight container in the refrigerator for about 3-4 days.

Nutrition Facts

Per serving (¼ of recipe) | Calories: 231 | Fat: 4g | Carbohydrates: 8g | Fiber: 3g | Sugars: 2g | Protein: 6g | Sodium: 114mg

Falafel

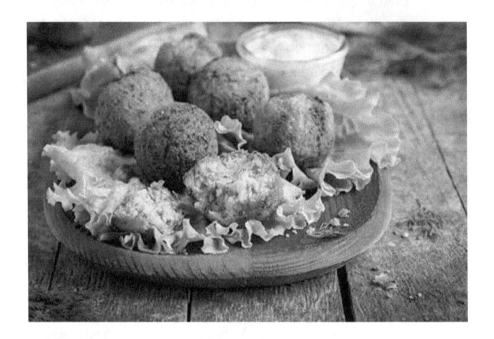

Preparation Time: 25 minutes + Soak Time (about 12 hours)

Cooking Time: 10-12 minutes

Yield: 18 falafel balls

Ingredients

- 1 cup dried chickpeas, soaked overnight (don't use canned chickpeas)
- ½ cup onion, roughly chopped
- 1 cup cilantro, roughly chopped (about a one large bunch)
- 1 cup parsley, roughly chopped (about a one large bunch)

- 3 garlic cloves
- 1 small green chile pepper, serrano or jalapeno pepper
- ½ teaspoon cardamom
- 1 teaspoon salt
- 1 teaspoon cumin
- ¼ teaspoon black pepper
- 2 tablespoons chickpea flour
- ½ teaspoon baking soda
- avocado oil for frying

Directions

1. The night before, put the chickpeas in a large bowl and cover them with cold water at least twice their volume. Leave to soak overnight, at least 12 hours.
2. The next day, drain the chickpeas. Place the drained, uncooked chickpeas in the bowl of a food processor. Add the onion, parsley, cilantro, pepper, garlic, cumin, salt, cardamom and black pepper to the food processor.
3. Pulse repeatedly, scraping down sides, until it is well-blended but still coarse like sand. Don't overwork it- this should not be smooth but rather quite coarse and granular.
4. Transfer the falafel mixture to a bowl and stir in the chickpea flour and baking soda. Then cover or add a lid. Refrigerate at least 30 minutes.

5. Scoop the falafel into 2 tablespoon-sized balls (a small ice cream scoop works well for this) and place on a parchment paper-lined baking sheet.
6. If you find the mixture is too wet, you can add another tablespoon of chickpea flour. If it's too dry and crumbly, you can add a teaspoon or two of water or lemon juice.
7. Fill a medium saucepan 3 inches with oil. Heat the oil on medium until it reaches 350°F.
8. Working in batches, carefully drop the falafel balls in the oil, about 6-8 at a time. Let them fry 1-3 minutes or so until golden brown.
9. Remove the cooked falafel to a paper towel-lined plate.
10. Serve the falafel immediately, while warm and crispy on the outside.

Nutrition Facts

Per serving (1 falafel ball) | Calories: 62 | Fat: 2g | Carbohydrates: 8g | Fiber: 2g | Sugars: 2g | Protein: 3g | Sodium: 170mg

One-Pan Roasted Salmon with Broccoli and Sweet Potatoes

Preparation Time: 10 minutes

Cooking Time: 25 minutes

Yield: 4 servings

Ingredients

- 2 sweet potatoes, peeled and cut into 1-inch cubes
- 12 ounces broccoli florets
- 4 salmon fillets (about 4-6 ounces each)
- 2 tablespoons olive oil, plus more for drizzling
- ¼ cup maple syrup
- 2 tablespoons Dijon mustard
- Salt and pepper

Directions

1. Heat oven to 425°F.
2. Line a rimmed baking sheet with aluminum foil and spray with cooking spray.
3. Toss broccoli, sweet potatoes and 2 tablespoons oil in large bowl to coat. Sprinkle with pinch of salt and pepper. Transfer to baking sheet.
4. Roast 10-15 minutes or until the potatoes are easily pierced with a fork.
5. While potatoes and broccoli are roasting, prepare glaze for salmon.

Combine maple syrup, mustard, $\frac{1}{4}$ teaspoon salt, and $\frac{1}{4}$ teaspoon pepper in a small bowl. Mix to combine.

6. Take the baking sheet out of the oven and turn oven setting to BROIL on "high."
7. Place salmon fillets in center of baking sheet. Space them $\frac{1}{2}$ inch apart, so they cook evenly. Arrange the vegetables around the salmon fillets. Coat top of salmon with the glaze.
8. Return the pan to the oven and broil 7-10 minutes or until fish flakes easily with fork and vegetables are tender. The total broiling time will depend on the size and thickness of your fish.
9. To serve, divide broccoli mixture and salmon between plates. Enjoy!

Nutrition Facts

Per serving ($\frac{1}{4}$ of the recipe) | Calories: 407 | Fat: 16g | Carbohydrates: 32g | Fiber: 4g | Sugars: 16g | Protein: 31g | Sodium: 213mg

One-Pan Sweet Potato Turkey

Preparation Time: 10 minutes

Cooking Time: 17-20 minutes

Yield: 4 servings

Ingredients

- 2 tablespoons extra virgin olive oil
- 1 pound free-range extra-lean ground turkey
- 1 teaspoon garlic clove, minced
- ½ cup onions, diced
- ½ cup yellow pepper, diced
- 1½ cups sweet potato, diced
- A pinch of salt and freshly ground black pepper
- A pinch of red chili flakes
- ½ cup shredded mozzarella cheese
- Fresh parsley, for garnishing

Directions

1. Pour the oil into a cast iron skillet and put the skillet over medium-high heat.
2. Once the oil is heated, add the ground turkey and garlic. Cook, breaking up meat with the side of a wooden spoon until meat is cooked through, about 5 minutes.

3. Add the onions and yellow peppers and cook until the onions are soft.
4. Add the sweet potato and red chili flakes; season with salt and pepper.
5. Cover the skillet and cook, stirring occasionally, until the sweet potatoes are tender.
6. Meanwhile, preheat the oven to 400°F.
7. When the sweet potatoes are tender, sprinkle the shredded mozzarella cheese over the top.
8. Transfer the skillet to the oven and bake until the cheese has melted, about 5 minutes.
9. Take the skillet out of the oven.
10. To serve, divide sweet potato mixture between plates; garnish with parsley.

Nutrition Facts

Per serving (¼ of the recipe) | Calories: 306 | Fat: 14g | Carbohydrates: 20g | Fiber: 3g | Sugars: 6g | Protein: 31g | Sodium: 186mg

Golden Lentil Curry

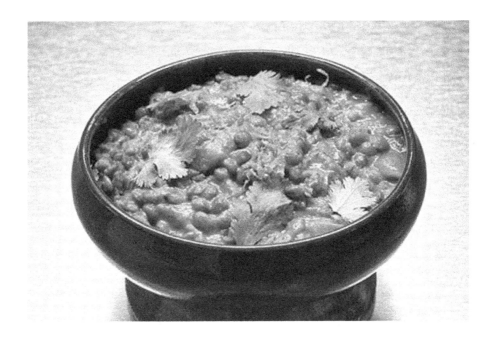

Preparation Time: 15 minutes + Soak Time (about 8 hours)

Cooking Time: 15 minutes

Yield: 6 servings

Ingredients

Lentils:

- 4 cups water
- 1½ cups golden (yellow) lentils, soaked overnight or for at least 8 hours, rinsed and drained

Coconut Curry Sauce:

- 1 tablespoon coconut oil
- 1 small shallot, diced (optional)
- 4 cloves garlic, minced
- 3 tablespoons fresh minced ginger
- 1 teaspoon ground turmeric
- ¾ teaspoon sea salt
- 1 heaping tablespoon curry powder
- ⅛ teaspoon cayenne pepper (for heat – omit if you don't like spice)
- 1¼-1½ cups light coconut milk
- 1-2 tablespoons coconut sugar or maple syrup(plus more to taste/or sub stevia)
- 2 tablespoons fresh lemon juice

Directions

1. Fill a large pot with water and bring it to a boil. Add lentils and bring back to a boil.
2. Turn heat down and simmer uncovered 4-5 minutes or until just tender. Then drain and set aside. Be sure not overcook your lentils because they can quickly turn into mush. For best results, follow the instructions on the package and pay attention to them as they cook.
3. Preheat a large rimmed skillet on medium heat for about 1-2 minutes. Once the pan is hot, add oil, shallot (optional), garlic, and ginger. Cook for 2-3 minutes, stirring frequently.

4. Season with salt, curry powder, turmeric, and cayenne and cook an additional 1 minute. Reduce the heat to low.
5. Stir in coconut milk and coconut sugar (or maple syrup) and cook over low heat for 3-4 minutes to combine the flavors.
6. Add the drained, cooked lentils to the coconut sauce and stir. Taste and adjust seasonings if needed.
7. Turn off heat, pour in lemon juice, and stir.
8. Serve and enjoy!

Nutrition Facts

Per serving (⅙ of recipe) | Calories: 102 | Fat: 5.1g | Carbohydrates: 11.9g | Fiber: 3g | Sugars: 2g | Protein: 3.9g | Sodium: 254mg

Cheesy Zucchini Squash Au Gratin

Preparation Time: 10 minutes

Cooking Time: 35 minutes

Yield: 4 servings

Ingredients

- 2 tablespoons butter
- ½ onion, thinly sliced
- 2 large cloves garlic, minced
- ½ cup heavy cream
- 1small zucchini, sliced in rounds ⅛ to ¼ inch thick
- 1small yellow squash, sliced in rounds ⅛ to ¼ inch thick
- ¼ cup parmesan
- 1 cup shredded smoked gouda

Directions

1. Preheat oven to 450°F.
2. Place butter pieces in an oven proof skillet. Cook over medium heat until the butter is melted, stirring occasionally with a wooden spoon.
3. Add the onions to the skillet. Cook 5 minutes or until the edges start to brown.
4. Stir in the minced garlic and cook 1 more minute.

5. Slowly pour the cream into the skillet and let it bubble up and thicken, about 2-3 minutes.
6. Slowly stir in parmesan. Add zucchini and yellow squash and continue to cook 4-5 more minutes.
7. Cover with the shredded gouda.
8. Place into oven and bake until cheese is golden brown, about 15-20 minutes.

Nutrition Facts

Per serving (¼ of recipe) | Calories: 247 | Fat: 20.2g | Carbohydrates: 11.1g | Sugars: 2.4g | Protein: 6.5g | Sodium: 215.2mg

One Skillet Mushroom Rice with Asparagus

Preparation Time: 10 minutes

Cooking Time: 15 minutes

Yield: 4 servings

Ingredients

- 1 tablespoon olive oil
- 2 garlic cloves, minced
- 2 cups mushroom, diced
- 1 cup asparagus (the spears should be cut at a diagonal in 1- and 2-inch pieces)
- 2 cups cooked rice
- 1 teaspoon fresh parsley, chopped
- 2 tablespoons feta cheese

Directions

1. Place a medium-sized skillet over medium-high heat and add olive oil. Once the oil is heated, add garlic and cook about 30 seconds until fragrant.
2. Stir in mushrooms and cook, uncovered and stirring occasionally, for about 5 minutes or until lightly browned and tender.
3. Add asparagus. Cook, stirring occasionally, about 3 to 4 minutes or until tender-crisp.
4. Stir in rice; season with salt and pepper. Cook about 2-3 minutes.

5. Garnish with fresh parsley. Sprinkle with feta cheese.
6. Serve and enjoy!

Nutrition Facts

Per serving (¼ of recipe) | Calories: 188 | Fat: 6g | Carbohydrates: 29g | Fiber: 2g | Sugars: 2g | Protein: 6g | Sodium: 114mg

Broccoli Soup

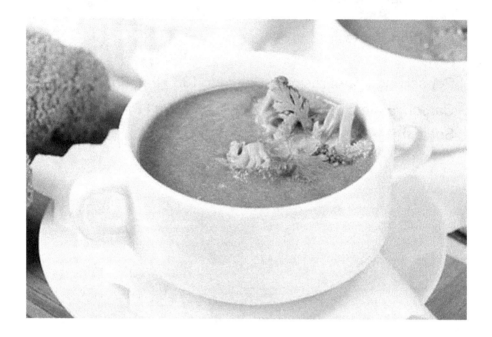

Preparation Time: 15 minutes

Cooking Time: 25-30 minutes

Yield: 8 servings

Ingredients

- 1½ teaspoons canola oil
- 1 large onion, diced
- 1 medium stalk celery, diced
- 1 clove garlic, minced
- 1 cup low-fat milk
- 2 (14½-ounce) cans low-sodium chicken broth

- 1 large potato, thinly sliced.
- 1 medium carrot, thinly sliced.
- 2 large broccoli crowns
- 1 whole bay leaf
- 1 ounce low-fat cheddar cheese, grated
- ¾ teaspoon salt
- ¼ teaspoon ground black pepper

Directions

1. Cut broccoli florets away from the stem. Slice stems thinly.
2. Place a large pot over medium-high heat and add canola oil. Once the oil is heated, add celery and onion. Cook about 6-8 minutes or until soft and lightly golden brown.
3. Stir in minced garlic and cook, stirring constantly, until fragrant, 30 seconds.
4. Pour milk and broth into the pot; add broccoli stems, potato, carrot and bay leaf to the mixture. Bring to a boil.
5. Turn the heat down to medium-low and simmer until veggies are soft, about 15 minutes. Add broccoli florets in the last 10 minutes.
6. Remove and discard bay leaf.
7. Carefully ladle half the soup into a blender* and process until smooth. Return purée to soup pot and stir in cheese, salt, and pepper. Stir over low heat until the cheese has melted.
8. To serve, ladle the soup into serving bowls.

*Note: Alternately, you can use a stick blender and puree the soup right in the cooking pot.

Nutrition Facts

Per serving (1½ cups) | Calories: 100 | Fat: 2.5g | Carbohydrates: 16g | Fiber: 2g | Sugars: 4g | Protein: 6g | Sodium: 320mg

Grilled Pork with Salsa

Preparation Time: 25 minutes + Marinating Time 2 hours

Cooking Time: 15 minutes

Yield: 6 servings

Ingredients

- 1-½ pounds pork tenderloin, cut into ¾-inch slices
- 2 tablespoons olive oil
- ½ cup lime juice
- ½ cup chopped sweet onion
- ¼ cup finely chopped seeded jalapeno peppers
- 4 teaspoons ground cumin
- 3 tablespoons jalapeno pepper jelly

Salsa:

- 2 plum tomatoes, seeded and chopped
- 2 medium ripe avocados, peeled and chopped
- 2 green onions, chopped
- 1 small cucumber, seeded and chopped
- 2 tablespoons minced fresh cilantro
- 1 tablespoon honey
- ¼ teaspoon salt
- ¼ teaspoon pepper

Directions

1. For marinade: In a bowl, whisk together the olive oil, lime juice, sweet onion, chopped jalapeno, and cumin. In a separate large bowl, add pork and ½ cup marinade; toss to coat. Cover and transfer to refrigerator for 2 hours.

2. For glaze: Add jelly and ⅓ cup of the remaining marinade to a small sauce pan and bring to a boil over medium-high heat. Cook, stirring occasionally, until slightly thickened, 1-2 minutes; remove from heat.

3. Place salsa ingredients in a large bowl; toss lightly with remaining marinade.

4. Remove pork from marinade, discarding marinade. Place pork on a lightly oiled grill rack over medium heat.

5. Cover and cook on grill until center registers 145°F on an instant read thermometer, about 4-5 minutes per side, brushing with glaze during the last 3 minutes.

6. Let rest off heat 3-5 minutes before serving.

7. Serve with salsa.

Nutrition Facts

Per serving (3 ounces cooked pork with ⅓ cup salsa) | Calories: 300 | Fat: 15g | Carbohydrates: 19g | Fiber: 4g | Sugars: 10g | Protein: 24g | Sodium: 155mg

Avocado Tuna Salad

Preparation Time: 5 minutes

Cooking Time: 0 minutes

Yield: 2 servings

Ingredients

- 1 (5 ounce) can wild albacore tuna, drained
- 1 small/medium avocado, peeled and pitted
- 2 tablespoons lemon juice
- 1 carrot, chopped
- 1 celery stalked, chopped
- ½ teaspoon dried dill weed
- ⅛ teaspoon smoked paprika
- 4 leafs romaine lettuce

Directions

1. In a medium bowl, flake the drained tuna with a fork. Add avocado to the tuna and mash with a fork, breaking up any large chunks.
2. Add the other ingredients and stir.
3. Chill 10-15 minutes.
4. Serve on a bed of fresh lettuce.

Nutrition Facts

Per serving (½ of recipe) | Calories: 240 | Fat: 15.6g | Carbohydrates: 12.9g | Fiber: 7.8g | Sugars: 2.6g | Protein: 16.2g | Sodium: 210.7mg

Quinoa Patties

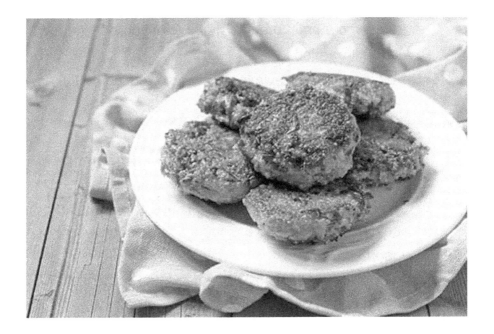

Preparation Time: 15 minutes

Cooking Time: from 45 minutes to 1 hour

Yield: 12 patties

Ingredients

- 2½ cups (or 12 oz.) cooked quinoa, at room temperature
- 4 large eggs, beaten
- ½ teaspoon fine-grain sea salt
- 1 yellow or white onion, finely chopped
- ⅓ cup freshly grated Parmesan or Gruyère cheese

- ⅓ cup finely chopped fresh chives
- 3 cloves garlic, finely chopped
- 1 cup whole grain bread crumbs, plus more if needed
- Water, if needed
- 1 tablespoon extra-virgin olive oil or clarified butter

Directions

1. Combine the quinoa, eggs, and salt in a medium bowl. Stir in the chives, onion, cheese, and garlic.
2. Stir the breadcrumbs into the mixture and let it stand about five minutes, so the liquid can be somewhat absorbed.
3. If the mixture seems overly wet, add an additional tablespoon of bread crumbs. If it seems too dry, add a tablespoon or two of water or broth.
4. Take small handfuls of the mixture and form into 12 little patties.
5. Place a large heavy skillet over medium low heat. Heat oil. Once the oil is heated, add patties to your skillet, being careful not to overload it so that you have trouble flipping the quinoa patties.
6. In 2 or 3 batches, cook the patties, covered, for 8-10 minutes on each side or until browned and golden.
7. If after 10 minutes your patties aren't brown, turn up the heat and cook (carefully to avoid burning) until they brown, about 5-7 minutes. Flip and cook for 5-7 more minutes on the other side.
8. Serve warm or at room temperature.

Nutrition Facts

Per serving (1 patty) | Calories: 111 | Fat: 4g | Carbohydrates: 13g | Fiber: 1g | Protein: 5g | Sodium: 158mg

Strawberry Almond Salad with Poppy Seed Dressing

Preparation Time: 10 minutes

Cooking Time: 0 minutes

Yield: 4 servings

Ingredients

For the dressing:

- 2 tablespoons olive oil
- 1½ tablespoons honey
- 1 tablespoon red wine vinegar
- 1 tablespoon cider vinegar
- ½ tablespoon poppy seeds
- 1 teaspoon minced shallots

For the salad:

- 5 oz. organic mixed baby greens
- 2 cups sliced strawberries
- ¼ cup slivered almond
- ¼ cup gorgonzola

Directions

1. In a large salad bowl, combine all the salad ingredients.

2. Add all the dressing ingredients to a mason jar and secure lid tightly.
3. Shake vigorously until ingredients are mixed thoroughly.
4. Pour over salad; gently toss to coat. Serve immediately.

Nutrition Facts

Per serving (¼ of recipe) | Calories: 198 | Fat: 14g | Carbohydrates: 16.5g | Fiber: 3.5g | Sugars: 12.5g | Protein: 5g | Sodium: 144.5mg

Fruity Peanut Butter Pockets

Preparation Time: 5 minutes

Cooking Time: 0 minutes

Yield: 2 servings

Ingredients

- 2 whole wheat pita pocket halves
- ¼ cup unsalted peanut butter
- ½ medium apple, thinly sliced
- ½ medium firm banana, sliced
- ⅛ teaspoon each ground allspice, cinnamon and nutmeg

Directions

1. In a small bowl, combine the unsalted peanut butter, allspice, cinnamon and nutmeg. Stir to combine all the ingredients.
2. Spread peanut butter mixture inside each half and divide apple and banana slices among pitas.
3. Enjoy!

Nutrition Facts

Per serving (1 pita half) | Calories: 324 | Fat: 17g | Carbohydrates: 36g | Fiber: 6g | Sugars: 13g | Protein: 12g | Sodium: 320mg

Baked Beet and Plum Salad

Preparation Time: 15 minutes

Cooking Time: about 1 hour 20 minutes

Yield: 6 servings

Ingredients

- 2 yellow bell peppers
- 4 golden beets (about 12 ounces)
- 8 yellow-fleshed plums, halved and pitted (about 1 pound)
- ½ pint yellow pear tomatoes, halved lengthwise
- ½ cup (2 ounces) crumbled goat cheese

For the vinaigrette:

- 2½ tablespoons extra-virgin olive oil
- 1 tablespoon white wine vinegar
- 1 tablespoon chopped fresh chives
- 1 teaspoon Dijon mustard
- 1 teaspoon chopped fresh thyme
- ¼ teaspoon salt
- ⅛ teaspoon freshly ground black pepper

Directions

1. Preheat broiler to high.

2. Cut the peppers in half lengthwise then remove the seeds and membranes. Lay the peppers on a foil-lined baking sheet, cut side down.
3. Broil for 13 minutes or until blackened. Place in a paper bag and fold tightly to seal. Set aside for 20 minutes.
4. Peel and slice bell peppers into ½-inch-thick strips.
5. Preheat oven to 450°F.
6. Leave root and 1-inch stem on beets; scrub with a brush. Add beets to an 11 x 7-inch ceramic or glass baking dish. Pour 1 inch of water into dish; cover tightly with foil.
7. Bake until beets can be pierced with a fork and are soft, 50 minutes to 1 hour depending on their size.
8. Let beets cool. Trim ends, peel skins, and slice into ½-inch-thick slices. Wearing gloves and working on parchment paper will minimize cleanup.
9. Combine all the ingredients for the vinaigrette in a small bowl, stirring well with a whisk.
10. Place sliced beets in a medium bowl. Pour 3 tablespoons vinaigrette over beets; toss gently. Let stand at least 15 minutes.
11. To serve, arrange the beets on 6 serving plates. Top each serving evenly with peppers, plums, and tomatoes.
12. Drizzle with remaining vinaigrette. Scatter over crumbled goat cheese.

Nutrition Facts

Per serving (⅙ of recipe) | Calories: 158 | Fat: 8g |
Carbohydrates: 20.2g | Fiber: 3.5g | Protein: 4.2g | Sodium:
194mg

Creamy Pumpkin Soup

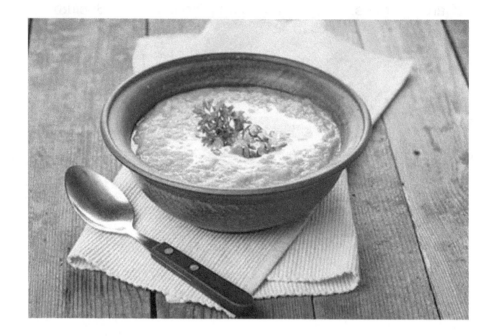

Preparation Time: 10 minutes

Cooking Time: 20 minutes

Yield: 7 cups

Ingredients

- 1 tablespoon olive oil
- 1 small onion, finely chopped
- 1 can (14 oz.) chicken broth
- 1 can (29 oz.) pumpkin
- 3 tablespoons brown sugar
- ¾ teaspoon curry powder
- 2 cups water

- ½ teaspoon salt
- 4 oz. (½ of 8-oz pkg.) Philadelphia Cream Cheese, cubed
- Ground nutmeg, optional

Directions

1. Place a large saucepan over medium heat and add olive oil. Once the oil is heated, add onion; cook, stirring occasionally, 3 minutes or until crisp-tender.
2. Stir in remaining ingredients except cream cheese until well-blended. Bring to boil. Turn the heat down to medium-low.
3. Add cream cheese; cook on medium-low, stirring constantly, for 3 to 5 minutes or until melted.
4. To serve, ladle the soup into serving bowls. Sprinkle each serving lightly with ground nutmeg, if desired.

Nutrition Facts

Per serving (1 cup) | Calories: 140 | Fat: 8g | Carbohydrates: 15g | Fiber: 4g | Sugars: 9g | Protein: 4g | Sodium: 420mg

Sheet Pan Roasted Chickpeas and Broccoli

Preparation Time: 10 minutes

Cooking Time: 20-25 minutes

Yield: 4 servings

Ingredients

- 1 (15-ounce) can chickpeas (garbanzo beans), drained, rinsed, and patted dry (I use no salt added or low salt versions)
- Olive oil cooking spray
- 3 to 4 cups broccoli florets
- 1 to 2 cups sugar snap peas
- 2 to 3 tablespoons olive oil
- ¼ to ⅓ cup nutritional yeast
- ¾ teaspoon kosher salt, or to taste
- ¾ teaspoon freshly ground black pepper, or to taste
- Fresh parsley, optional for garnishing

Directions

1. Preheat oven to 400°F.
2. On a baking sheet lined with aluminum foil, spread chickpeas in a single layer then spray them with cooking spray and bake about 15 minutes.
3. Take the baking sheet out of the oven. Add the broccoli, sugar snap peas, evenly drizzle everything

236

with olive oil, evenly sprinkle the nutritional yeast, salt, pepper, and toss with your hands to coat evenly.
4. Roast 10-12 minutes until broccoli is cooked through (check by poking with a fork, should be fork tender) and lightly browned.
5. Garnish with parsley if desired.

Nutrition Facts

Per serving (¼ of recipe) | Calories: 274 | Fat: 10g | Carbohydrates: 35g | Fiber: 12g | Sugars: 7g | Protein: 15g | Sodium: 255mg

Pistachio-Crusted Baked Fish

Preparation Time: 15 minutes

Cooking Time: 15-20 minutes

Yield: 4 servings

Ingredients

- 4 (4-5 ounce) fresh or frozen trout fillets
- ½ teaspoon caraway seeds
- ½ teaspoon coriander seeds
- ½ teaspoon cumin seeds
- 4 teaspoons olive oil
- 1 clove garlic, minced
- 1 teaspoon finely shredded lemon peel
- ¼ teaspoon ground cinnamon
- ¼ teaspoon ground pepper
- ½ teaspoon kosher salt
- ¼ cup pistachio nuts, finely chopped
- 4 lemon wedges

Directions

1. Thaw fish if frozen. Preheat oven to 350°F. Line a shallow baking pan with foil and coat with cooking spray.

2. To toast seeds, place them in a small saucepan on low heat and stir frequently for three to four minutes. Don't walk too far away while you are toasting the seeds, since they can go from perfect to burned very quickly.
3. Remove from heat. Transfer seeds to a small food processor or a mortar and pestle and grind them. Add oil, lemon peel, garlic, cinnamon, pepper, and salt. Stir to combine.
4. Add pistachios to a small bowl; set aside.
5. Rinse fish under cold running water and pat dry with paper towels.
6. Spread one side of the fish fillets with the spice mixture. Bringing up two opposite ends, fold the fish into thirds. Dip the top and the sides of the fish bundles into the nuts to coat; place in the prepared baking pan. Scatter with any remaining nuts.
7. Bake 15-20 minutes or until fish flakes easily with fork.
8. Then garnish with lemon wedges and serve.

Nutrition Facts

Per serving (1 crusted fish fillet) | Calories: 227 | Fat: 12g | Carbohydrates: 4g | Fiber: 1g | Sugars: 1g | Protein: 25g | Sodium: 283mg

The Mediterranean Diet Guide:

14-Day Meal Plan Including 42 Quick and Awesome Recipes

By

Stephanie N. Collins

Introduction

In the busy world we live in today, fast foods, junk foods, and low-priced meat are gaining popularity. Why? Because they are easier and quicker to cook. You don't have to be a renowned chef to cook instant noodles or microwave pre-cooked store-bought meals. Unfortunately, the majority of the population prefers quick meals to quality food. This is mostly due to the fast-paced world we live in; everyone is on a hurry to make ends meet and get on with their lives. Eating is no longer a pleasurable experience that nourishes your body and soul; it is now a means of survival.

Before you go out and restock your cupboards with instant ramen, what if I told you there is a healthier alternative? Cooking healthy doesn't necessarily need to take an entire day of preparation. You do not have to sacrifice your productivity for the day to enjoy a nice hefty meal. Without sacrificing your time, you can quickly whip up a nutritional meal for you and your loved ones, whether you're searching for a budget friendly meal you can whip up in your dorm room or a nice meal for the family after a nerve wrecking Friday night.

Doesn't a meal cooked in olive oil, wine, and wheat sound mouthwatering? Then you'd be glad to hear about the Mediterranean cuisine. These dishes have French, Egyptian, Greek, Turkish, and Spanish influences. These countries surround the Mediterranean Sea, which explains where the name came from. They include ingredients and processes known to this region. In recent studies, the Mediterranean cuisine has proved to be a good diet plan for heart care and losing weight.

The Mediterranean diet is filled with healthy fats that help keep your brain active, and it is known to reduce the risk of heart diseases. This diet is perfect for people on the go and those who are health conscious. It is also a healthy alternative to untested modern diets. A key ingredient to the Mediterranean diet is to eat lots of fruits, vegetables and healthy fats as often as possible. And it doesn't have to be a budget-crushing meal because there are many ways to substitute ingredients.

Mediterranean dishes are jam packed with the nutrients you need on a day-to-day basis. You might argue that it's too expensive or it will take too much of your time, but that is where you are wrong. There are ways to cut down on your expenses without sacrificing nutrients or food quality. For example, you can substitute canned fish for fresh, peanuts for other nuts and seeds; you can also replace meat or fish with whole grains. It is also good practice to purchase dry goods in bulk. When you're in the produce section, keep an open mind for fruits and vegetables on sale. You can also opt for frozen food variants.

Having a balanced diet can still be fun and budget friendly, especially with the Mediterranean diet. You don't have to break the bank to enjoy a delicious and nutritious meal. To top that all off, this diet is quick and easy to make, and it will be your loved one's favorite.

Chapter 1: Everything You Need to Know about The Mediterranean Diet

The Mediterranean cuisine is as colorful and flavorful as the rich culture it represents. Several countries that surround the Mediterranean Sea have a significant influence on the popular cuisine. Today, many follow the Mediterranean diet not only for its mouth-watering dishes but also for the health benefits that come along with it.

This cuisine originated in the Mediterranean basin, known as "the cradle of society". Imagine a convergence zone of all the history of the ancient world, which is the Mediterranean basin. This is where cultures from all over the world planted their roots and is also why their influence on food is so widespread.

We can divide the Mediterranean Diet into two words. By doing so, we can further understand the rich history of the classic cuisine. In the 3rd century, Solinos coined the term "Mare Mediterraneum", which translates to *the sea between two continents*. The Mediterranean Sea is between Europe, Asia, and Africa. The bountiful sea was the main source of delicacies in the early centuries, and as a convergence zone for travelers, seafarers, and foreign merchants, the culture of the neighboring countries was easily spread and passed on. On the other hand, "Diet" comes from the Latin word "Daita", which means 'way of living'. Now you see, the Mediterranean diet is not just a way to eat but also a way of life. It is a habit that must be followed should you want to get all the benefits that have been perfected through the ages.

In the early 1940s and 1950s, the Mediterranean diet first gained popularity. During this time in history, many were seeking healthier options that could give them all the nutrition they needed for the day without risking their productivity. These diets focus on maintaining a healthy amount of proteins, carbs, fat, and other nutrients you need to maintain a healthy lifestyle. Rest assured that following the Mediterranean diet will make your body nutritionally sound with a wide array of foods and flavors without putting in too much time preparing and cooking your meals. Most of the recipes are easy to follow no matter how experienced you are in cooking, and to make it better, the ingredients can be found in your local store.

The Mediterranean diet ranks the number 1 best diet over all, number 17 in the best weight-loss diet, and number 1 in the best diets for diabetics. So, if you're health conscious but still want to enjoy a variety of flavors, switch over to the Mediterranean diet today.

Did you know that those who live near the Mediterranean Sea live a healthier and longer life far from cancer and cardiovascular illnesses compared to those in most of America? Don't be surprised, because this diet has low red meat and saturated fat. You might argue that Greek food is on the opposite side of the spectrum, far from French or Turkish; you are correct, but they follow the same principles. By exploring the Mediterranean Diet pyramid, we'll get a better glimpse on how to abide by the diet and plan your meals accordingly.

Chapter 2: Mediterranean Diet Pyramid

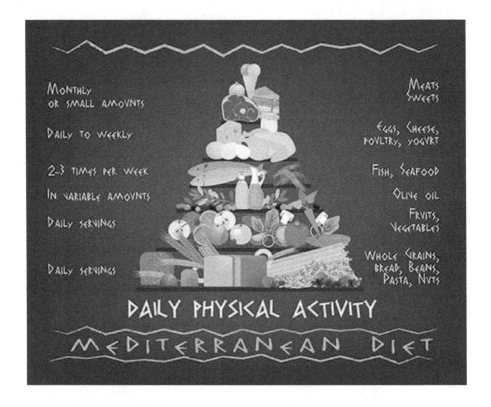

In 1993, Old ways together with Harvard School of Public Health and the World Health Organization gave the world the "Mediterranean Diet Pyramid". This was published to guide us through the right consumption of food and the frequency of what we should include in our meal plans.

As you can see, the building block of this diet is physical activity. A proper diet is meant to help you have a healthy lifestyle, which means eating nutritious food while being physically active. If you're working to be physically fit, just eating right is not enough. You have to put in as much work on your body as the food you are eating. But exercise doesn't mean you have to go to the gym every day. You would be happy to know that even walking at a leisurely pace can work wonders on your health. By walking 20-30 minutes a day, you are increasing the strength of your heart and lungs, fortifying your bones and muscles, and enjoying your daily dose of endorphins. You can also do a few squats before starting your day or plank for a minute daily. Small but consistent efforts of physical activity give your body a huge boost in the right direction.

On a daily basis, you should consume more fruits, vegetables, and healthy fats multiple times a day. Legumes, like beans and peas, unrefined whole grain such as brown rice, and steel cutouts should be consumed at least once a day. These are the foundations of the Mediterranean diet; they are natural and organic means of nutrition. Not only do they contain most of the nutrients you need to keep your body healthy and productive, but they are also easily prepared and bought. And if you are mindful of your carbon emissions or just want to try your hand at gardening, you are in luck. Most of these foods can be easily grown in your own backyard. Beans, beets, bell peppers, and leafy greens are some of the vegetables you can easily grow in your backyard. You can also try using hydroponics to grow tomatoes, cucumbers, spring onions, spinach, and even berries.

Fish and seafood should be part of your diet multiple times a week. These are excellent alternatives to getting your dose of protein. They are low fat, making it easier to maintain your diet. Fish has high levels of Omega-3, which are good for your heart and brain. They are also perfect for expecting and nursing mothers, since fish has nutrients that aid in the development of the brain and eyes. The American Heart Association also encourages people to eat at least 2 servings of non-fried fish in a week. Fish is abundant in nutrients that your body needs. In a recent study by the American Medical Associate (JAMA), consuming fish regularly helps maintain a good memory and reduces the risk of Alzheimer's disease by up to 47%. Fish is also a great way to fend off inflammation; due to its richness in Omega-3, they can reduce symptoms of rheumatoid arthritis and reduce the need for artificial painkillers. Over 70 million people suffer from high blood pressure; however, by maintaining fish in your diet, you won't encounter problems in regulating your cholesterol levels.

Chicken, eggs, and organic cheese and yogurt should be limited to 3-4 times a month. Chicken is also a great source of protein, carbohydrates, vitamins and minerals. However, it also comes with calories and saturated fat; the breast or the white meat is a healthier alternative. Eggs, on the other hand, contain Vitamin D that is necessary for good bone structure, choline that's needed for normal bodily function, lutein and antioxidants that reduce the risk of developing cataracts. Yogurts are high in probiotics, which help your digestive system work as it should, processing all the nutrients and flushing out the toxins. With all the nutrients you can get from these ingredients, they also come with a few health risks such as cholesterol. That is why they should be consumed a few times a month; that way you can reap all the goodness of their nutrients without risking your health and diet.

Most of all, you should rarely indulge in saturated fat from red meat and dairy, refined sugars, and deli meats. It is good to allow yourself a cheat day once in a while but always keep meals in proper portion. Too much of anything will always be bad for you.

Chapter 3: 8 Reasons to Start your Mediterranean Diet Today

The traditional Mediterranean diet is known to reduce the risk of heart disease due to low levels of "bad" cholesterol build-up. It is also known to reduce the risk of cancer, Parkinson's, and Alzheimer's disease. Maintaining a Mediterranean diet is known to:

1. Boost and Preserve Memory.

The Mediterranean diet is filled with healthy fats that prevent dementia and dullness of cognitive functions while boosting memory and brainpower. By following a Mediterranean diet, you are sure to have a sharp mind and healthy body.

In a study released by the American Medical Association's JAMA Internal Medicine, it showed that elderly participants that followed the Mediterranean diet, specifically olive oil and nuts, counteract age-related dullness of the mind.

2. Lessen the Risk of Heart Disease.

Studies also show that, when the diet is maintained, it can drastically lower the risks of cardiovascular diseases, such as coronary heart disease, myocardial infarction, and stroke. This is because the Mediterranean diet promotes "good" cholesterol and healthy fats that do not clog up your arteries, ensuring healthy and consistent blood flow.

3. Helps Strengthen Bones.

It shouldn't come as a shock to know that the Mediterranean diet helps keep your bones strong and healthy. Compounds in olive oil help your bone cells mature, which leads to sturdier bone structure and quicker recovery time for bone injuries. It is also known to prevent osteoporosis.

4. Controls Blood Sugar & Helps Manage Diabetes.

If you're struggling to keep your blood sugar in check, then the Mediterranean diet is something you should try today. This diet has been proven very beneficial for those struggling with diabetes. The diet promotes including naturally sweet nuts like almonds, walnuts, and pistachios, which you can substitute for sweet pastries.

5. Fight Depression.

In 2013, a study found that adhering to the Mediterranean diet helps control depression. Consuming fresh produce like lentils and nuts can signal your brain to produce endorphins that make you feel lighter and happier.

6. Make Weight Loss Feel Like a Breeze.

Since the diet promotes healthy fat and "good" cholesterol, you won't have any problems controlling your weight. Consumption of meat and trans-fat from margarine, milk, cheese, and yogurt is limited to special occasions or a few times a month.

7. Wine! Wine! Wine!

One of the key ingredients to Mediterranean cuisine is wine. Enjoying alcohol in moderation is known to reduce the risk of heart diseases. This diet usually moderates wine consumption to 5 to 10 ounces a day. Red wine is also a great way to raise levels of Omega-3 fatty acids, which are good for the heart.

8. A Longer Happier Life.

Including whole foods and leafy greens in your diet will keep your body healthy and active. Partner it with the right exercise and you greatly reduce your mortality rate by 20%.

Chapter 4: Do's and Don'ts of The Mediterranean Diet

If it is your first time trying a diet plan, it might seem difficult and daunting at first. You really have to put all effort in maintaining a healthy lifestyle and not abusing your cheat days. Let's lay out some easy to follow ground rules on the Do's and Don'ts of following the Mediterranean diet.

Include fruits like berries and citrus fruits in your meal plans every day. Berries are full of antioxidants that control free radicals in your body. They also improve insulin levels and help maintain adequate amounts of blood sugar. They are high in fiber and fight inflammation. Not only do they lower your bad cholesterol levels, but they also are very beneficial for your skin. Citrus fruits, on the other hand, are great sources of Vitamin C, which is something you need especially during flu seasons. Citrus fruits are also great for your heart since they are rich in antioxidants that help people recover and keep your immune system secured.

Have a portion of vegetables and legumes in your everyday diet. Legumes, like kidney beans, soybeans, chickpeas, and lentils, are excellent sources of fiber and protein that you need to keep your body healthy and active. They are also very rich in Vitamin B, iron, zinc, magnesium, and antioxidants.

Eat more grains, such as whole wheat and fiber products, in your meal plans. Oatmeal, flaxseed, and Buckwheat are not only high in fiber but also lower the risks of heart problems. They are also rich sources of Vitamin B, selenium, magnesium, and iron. By selecting whole grains, you can rest easy knowing you're getting all the nutrients you need while being able to maintain your weight and a healthy diet easily.

Include some nuts especially walnuts and almonds. There is a common misconception that nuts are bad for you. That cannot be farther from the truth. In recent years, studies have found that nuts, such as almonds, cashews, walnuts, pecans, and even peanuts, are great alternatives to getting your daily dose of nutrients. Almonds have the highest calcium content compared to other nuts. They are also rich in fiber, Vitamin E, and magnesium that help lower bad cholesterol levels. Cashews and hazelnuts are iron rich and have the same unsaturated fat content as olive oil. Walnuts are perfect for taking care of your heart since they contain high levels of Omega-3 and antioxidants that keep your brain active and your body free of cancer. Did you know that Peanuts are considered legumes? That is because of the high folate percentage of these nuts that make them perfect for brain development especially during pregnancy.

Use olive oil instead of butter. Olive oil has high levels of Omega-6 and Omega-3 fatty acids that work wonders for your heart. They also contain antioxidants that may reduce chronic disease risks; it decreases the chances of having a stroke and has high anti-inflammatory properties. The best part is that by substituting your oil with Olive oil, you lower your risks of diabetes, cancer, and even Alzheimer's.

A glass of red wine works wonders. In the early centuries, wine would often be used to treat health conditions. To this day, we still keep up with this practice. Moderate consumption of red wine has proven to increase life expectancy. Why? Red wine has a compound known as *resveratrol*, which is a natural compound produced by plants to ward off bacteria, fungi, and protect from ultraviolet radiation. Resveratrol is secreted by the skin of grapes when processed to make red wine, and blueberries and cranberries are excellent sources of this compound. Red wine improves your heart health by raising Omega-3 levels of fatty acid that makes sure your blood vessels are doing their job. By drinking a glass a day, you can rest assured that you are keeping your heart and brain healthy and in check. But remember, always drink in moderation. Enjoying a glass of red wine is great for your body; a bottle of red wine doesn't have the same effect.

Don't include sugar in your diet. Sugar is everywhere. Yes, it is difficult to avoid, but it is something you should be very wary about. In recent years, more and more of the population are becoming obese. The prime suspect to this health crisis is SUGAR. It might taste good, but it is very bad for your body. Sugar causes your glucose levels to be irregular, hence you might suffer from mood swings, fatigue, and headaches. They also contribute largely to obesity, diabetes, and heart disease. To make matters worse, high blood sugar decreases the effectiveness of your immune system. This is because bacteria and yeast thrive on sugar, therefore making you vulnerable to diseases.

Limit your consumption of red meat. Enjoying a nice juicy steak might seem tempting, but according to the World Health Organization (WHO), red meat is considered carcinogenic. Red meats have high concentrations of saturated fat that raises the level of bad cholesterol in your body. They also have high levels of LDL that put you at risk of heart disease. And deli meat or processed meat is 10 times worse than red meat. No matter how lean or grade a meat you consume, they still pose the same threats. But consuming them once in a while, especially during special occasions, is okay. You can also counter the harmful effects of eating red meat by maintaining a healthy diet.

Chapter 5: Lifestyle and The Mediterranean Diet

People often associate dieting with merely eating fewer carbs and losing weight. But dieting takes so much more than that. The Mediterranean diet isn't just about losing or maintaining weight; it is about the improvement of one's lifestyle in general. This is why the foundations of this diet are activities and exercise. It aims to be a guide for you to achieve a positive and healthy lifestyle holistically.

A study published in 2009 by the Journal of the American Medical Association (JAMA) found that those who observe the Mediterranean diet had lower risks of cognitive decline; the same journal also found that, if the diet is paired with physical activities, it is a more effective way to reduce the risk of Dementia and Alzheimer's. You might be thinking you have to hit the gym for the diet to reach its full potential; that is where you are wrong. You can choose a rigorous workout or participate in light physical activities. Doing so can reduce the risks of cognitive decline.

Because the Mediterranean diet is a holistic approach, it is best paired not only with physical activities but with mental stimulation as well. A study by Almudena Sanchez-Villegas shows the link between the Mediterranean diet and reducing the risk of depression. The Mediterranean lifestyle focuses not only on eating right but also productive socialization. Maintaining a significant volume of positive social connections in a week can boost your mood and lower your blood pressure.

With all that being said, merely dieting is never enough. One must always strive to have a healthy mind, body, and spirit.

Chapter 6: 14 Days Meal Plan

In this cookbook, there are 14 recipes for breakfast, lunch, and dinner, respectively. This is to help you ease into the transition of adhering to the Mediterranean diet.

We always plan our activities for the day, so why not include your meals? By creating your meal plan, you will not only be able to budget your expenses, but you can save time as well.

Let's talk about the five benefits of Meal Plans.

1. Portion Control.

Having a meal plan will let you see how much you are eating daily. It would be easier for you to know whether you are overeating. It is also an excellent way for you not to cook more than you can eat. Learning how to control meal portions is a step forward in having a healthy lifestyle.

2. Healthy Eating.

Because of a meal plan, you won't be inclined to walk over to the nearest fast-food joint. You will be able to eliminate any trouble with having a balanced diet.

3. Time Management.

Have you ever been hungry and realize there's nothing in the fridge? Or stressing over what to cook for the day and realize you don't have enough ingredients? All of this can be avoided with a meal plan. Since you have mapped out your menu for the week, you can stop by the store and pick up some ingredients. It would also be easier for you to allot time in your day for cooking a healthy meal because you know exactly how long your meal preparation and cooking times are going to be.

4. Budget Saver.

We all want to save money, and meal planning is the ticket to it. By properly planning out what meals you will be eating for the day, you can budget how much each meal will cost. It is also more cost effective if you can see similar ingredients for different meals, so you can buy in bulk. Having a detailed list of your meals keeps you from impulse buying and over buying.

5. No More Food Waste.

Your meal plan will make sure you buy ingredients with a purpose and not buy excessively. Gone are the days when you stack your fridge with expiring ingredients because you were unable to use them. This also works perfectly for those that are eco-friendly and want to live a zero-waste lifestyle.

Chapter 7: Easy Mediterranean Diet Recipes

The Mediterranean diet is all about eating whole foods, beans, olive oil, and a lot of fruits and vegetables. It limits the intake of processed foods and saturated fat, which makes it a great way to combat cardiovascular diseases and diabetes. This diet doesn't have a lot of Do's and Don'ts but focuses more on eating as many heart-healthy foods as you can. It is more sustainable than other strict diets.

Because the Mediterranean diet is based on fresh produce, professionals often give the impression that it is difficult to cook and takes too much of your time. On the contrary, this diet is relatively easy to prepare, with most of the recipes only needing one pan and a few steps. Anyone with as little as no cooking experience to seasoned professionals can prepare a healthy Mediterranean meal.

You might not have been used to following a diet or having meal plans but don't let it prevent you from starting to live healthier. By following these 42 quick and easy recipes, you'll be reaping all the benefits of the Mediterranean diet in no time.

Mediterranean Breakfast Ideas

Barley with Mixed Vegetable Salad

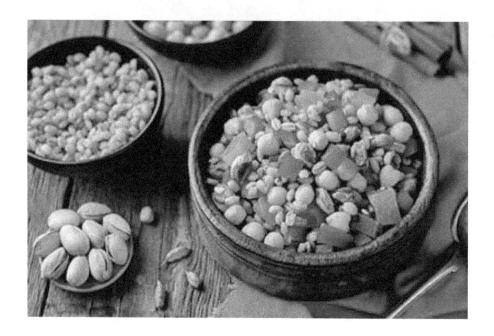

Preparation Time: 15 minutes

Cooking Time: 45 minutes

Yields: 4 servings

Ingredients

- 1 cup arugula leaves
- 3 tablespoons sun-dried tomatoes, packed without oil (finely chopped)
- 1 cup pearl barley (uncooked)

- 1 (15½-ounce) can unsalted chickpeas (rinsed and drained)
- 1 cup red bell pepper (finely chopped)
- 2 tablespoons extra-virgin olive oil
- 2 tablespoons Fresh lemon juice
- ½ teaspoon crushed red pepper
- 2 tablespoons pistachios (chopped)
- 1 teaspoon salt

Directions

1. Begin by cooking your barley according to package instructions, omitting salt.
2. Transfer the cooked barley to a large bowl and combine it with arugula, tomatoes, chickpeas, and bell pepper. Set aside.
3. In a separate bowl combine lemon juice, extra-virgin olive oil, pepper, and salt. Thoroughly whisk to combine.
4. Now, get your bowl of barley mixture and drizzle it with the lemon juice mixture.
5. Garnish with a sprinkle of pistachios.

Nutrition Facts

Per serving (1¼ cups barley mixture and 1½ teaspoons pistachios) | Calories: 359 | Total Fat: 10g | Saturated Fat: 1g | Monounsaturated Fat: 5g | Carbohydrates: 61g | Sugar: 3g | Sodium: 852mg | Fiber: 14g | Protein 11g

Mediterranean Baked Halibut

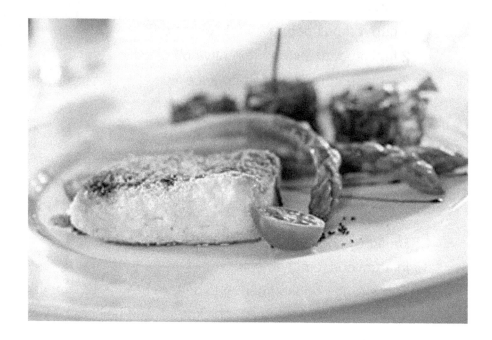

Preparation Time: 10 minutes

Cooking Time: 15 minutes

Yield: 6 servings

Ingredients

For the Sauce:

- Zest of 2 lemons
- Juice of 2 lemons
- 1 cup Greek extra-virgin olive oil
- 1½ tablespoons garlic (minced)
- 2 teaspoons dill weed

- 1 teaspoon seasoned salt
- ½ teaspoon black pepper
- 1 teaspoon dried oregano
- ½ teaspoon ground coriander

For the Fish:

- 1 pound fresh green beans
- 1 pound cherry tomatoes
- 1 large yellow onion (sliced into half-moons)
- 1½ pounds halibut fillet (sliced into 1½-inch pieces)

Directions

1. Start by preheating your oven to 425°F.
2. Meanwhile, add all the sauce ingredients to a large mixing bowl and whisk together.
3. Add the green beans, tomatoes, and onions. Toss to coat with sauce evenly. Spread the vegetables on one side of baking sheet in a single layer.
4. Add the halibut fillet strips to the sauce and coat evenly. Place on the other side of baking sheet and pour the remaining sauce mixture on top.
5. Sprinkle lightly with more seasoned salt. Bake in preheated oven for 15 minutes then broil for 3 minutes.
6. It is best to enjoy with a salad or brown rice.

Nutrition Facts

Per serving (⅙ of recipe) | Calories: 649 | Fat: 32.9g |
Saturated Fat: 5.1g | Carbohydrates: 57.3g | Sugar: 0.4g |
Sodium: 107.5mg | Protein: 31.8g

Greek Style Quinoa Dish with Veggies

Preparation Time: 10 minutes

Cooking Time: 20 minutes

Yields: 6 breakfast bowls

Ingredients

- 12 eggs
- ¼ cup plain Greek yogurt
- 1 teaspoon onion powder
- 1 teaspoon granulated garlic
- ½ teaspoon of salt
- ½ teaspoon of pepper
- 1 teaspoon olive oil
- 5 ounces baby spinach
- 1 pint cherry tomatoes
- 1 cup feta cheese
- 2 cups cooked quinoa

Directions

1. Whisk eggs, Greek yogurt, onion powder, granulated garlic, salt, and pepper together. Set aside.
2. Heat olive oil in a skillet and add baby spinach. Cook baby spinach for 3-4 minutes or until slightly wilted.
3. Add cherry tomatoes and cook until softened.

4. Add egg mixture and cook, stirring frequently, 7-9 minutes.
5. When your eggs are set, add the feta cheese and quinoa. Cook until heated through.

Nutrition Facts

Per serving (1¼ cups) | Calories: 357g | Fat: 20g | Saturated fat: 8g | Carbohydrates: 20g | Fiber: 3g | Protein: 23g

Egg Muffins with Ham

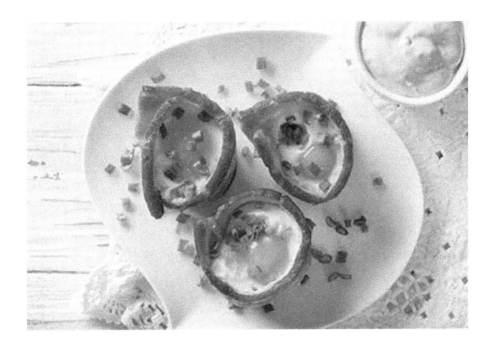

Preparation Time: 10 minutes

Cooking Time: 15 minutes

Yield: 6 Egg Muffins

Ingredients

- 9 slices of thin cut ham
- ½ cup canned roasted red bell pepper (sliced for further garnish)
- ⅓ cup French spinach (minced)
- ¼ cup Feta cheese (crumbled or grated)
- 5 large eggs

- Pinch of salt and pepper
- 1½ tablespoons. of Pesto sauce
- Fresh Basil as garnish

Directions

1. First, preheat your oven to 400°F.
2. Spray muffin tins with cooking spray to prevent the muffins from sticking after baking.
3. Line each muffin tin with 1 and a half pieces of ham; make sure there are no holes for your egg mixture to leak out. Place a little bit of roasted red bell pepper on the bottom of each muffin tin. Place 1 tablespoon of minced spinach on top of the red bell pepper. Top with ½ tablespoon of crumbled Feta cheese.
4. Break the eggs into a bowl, whisk, adding salt and pepper. Pour the beaten eggs into each muffin tin.
5. Bake the muffins for 15-17 minutes until all the eggs are puffy.
6. Take the muffin tins out of the oven. Garnish each muffin with ¼ teaspoon of pesto sauce, additional roasted red bell pepper, and freshly sliced basil.

Nutrition Facts

Per serving (1 egg muffin) | Calories: 109 | Fat: 6.7g | Saturated Fat: 2.4g | Carbohydrates: 1.8g | Sugar: 1.2g | Sodium: 423mg | Fiber: 1.8g | Protein 9.3g

Watermelon and Cheese Salad

Preparation Time: 10 minutes

Yield: 4 servings

Ingredients

- 8 ounces of halloumi cheese (cut into ½-inch cubes)
- ½ cup of black olives (pitted and halved)
- 1 cup packed fresh green za'atar leaves (or substitute with a fresh thyme, oregano, and a touch of marjoram)
- 2 shallots (diced)
- 1 tablespoon sumac
- Juice of 1 lemon
- Juice of 1 lime
- 6 tablespoons of olive oil
- ½ teaspoon fresh chili, such as jalapeno (finely diced)
- Sea salt
- 3 pounds of watermelon (seeded and cut into 1-inch cubes)
- 1 cup seedless grapes
- 1 large cucumber (peeled and coarsely chopped)

Directions

1. In a large bowl, mix cheese, olives, za'atar, shallots, sumac, lemon juice, lime juice, oil, and chili then season with salt.

2. Place watermelon, grapes, cucumber, and cheese mixture in a serving bowl. Gently mix well.

Nutrition Facts

Per serving (¼ of recipe) | Calories: 581 | Fat: 41.9g | Saturated Fat: 15.5g | Carbohydrates: 41.4g | Sugar: 29.1g | Sodium: 840mg | Fiber: 4.2g | Protein 17.9g

Mediterranean Tuna Melt Sandwiches

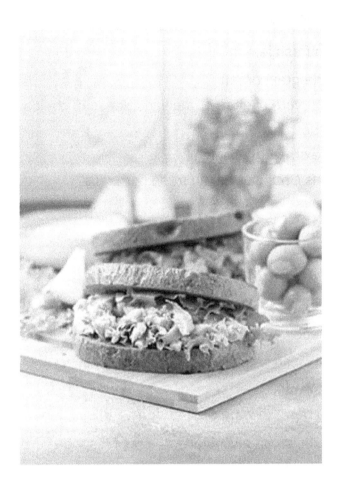

Preparation Time: 10 minutes

Cooking Time: 10 minutes

Yield: 4 Tuna Melt sandwiches

Ingredients

- 10 ounces canned tuna in oil (drained)

- ¼ red onion (diced)
- ½ cup cucumber yogurt Tzatziki
- ½ teaspoon fresh lemon juice
- 8 slices whole-grain bread
- 4 slices of Gruyere cheese or melting cheese of choice
- 4 leaves lettuce or romaine
- 1 teaspoon extra-virgin olive oil
- 2 tablespoons Chopped mixed fresh herbs (Dill, parsley, or mint)
- Salt and pepper to taste
- 1 avocado

Directions

1. Cut an avocado in half and remove the pit. Remove the avocado flesh with a spoon and slice into ¼-inch thick slices. Set aside.
2. In a medium bowl, mix the drained tuna and cucumber yogurt. Add the diced red onions and ¼ teaspoon lemon juice. Fold everything gently to let the flavors blend.
3. Preheat the broiler or oven toaster. Toast the slices of whole-grain bread under the broiler. Remove four slices and set aside. Top each remaining bread slice with one slice of cheese and toast in the oven for 1 to 3 minutes or until the cheese has fully melted.

4. In another bowl, whisk olive oil and ¼ teaspoon of lemon juice. Add in the greens and herbs. Toss everything with a dash of salt and pepper.
5. Layer the salad, tuna, and avocado on 4 pieces of plain bread and top with the toasted cheese slices, cheese side down. Cut diagonally and enjoy!

Nutrition Facts

Per serving (1 portion) | Calories: 599 | Fat: 28.8g | Saturated Fat: 10g | Carbohydrates: 50.9g | Sugar: 9.4g | Sodium: 767mg | Fiber: 13.7g | Protein 26.9g

Red Pepper-Walnut Spread

Preparation Time: 15 minutes

Cooking Time: 30 minutes (not including overnight chilling)

Yield: 3 cups of spread

Ingredients

- 2½ pounds of sweet red bell peppers
- 1 small hot chili pepper or 1 tablespoon of Turkish red pepper paste
- 1½ cups of walnuts
- ½ cup wheat crackers
- 1 tablespoon of lemon juice
- 2 tablespoons pomegranate molasses
- ½ teaspoon ground cumin
- Salt to taste
- ½ teaspoon of sugar
- 2 tablespoons olive oil

Directions

1. Start by roasting the peppers and chili over a gas burner or broiler until blacked for about 12 minutes.
2. Place in a bowl and cover with plastic wrap and let steam for 10 minutes. Remove the skin and the stems. Transfer to plate lined with paper towels; let drain for 10 minutes.

3. Using a food processor, grind the walnuts and crackers with lemon juice, pomegranate molasses, cumin, salt, and sugar until smooth and pasty. Add the peppers and process until pureed. With the motor running, pour in the olive oil. Cover and transfer to the refrigerator overnight.
4. Bring to room temperature before serving and sprinkle with cumin and olive oil.
5. You can use the spread on whole-grain loaves for a quick and healthy breakfast to start your day.

Nutrition Facts

Per serving (2 tablespoons) | Calories: 89 | Fat: 6.4g | Saturated Fat: 0.7 g | Carbohydrates: 6.7g | Sugar: 3.3 g | Sodium: 7.7 mg | Fiber: 1.6g | Protein 1.9 g

Zucchini Quiche

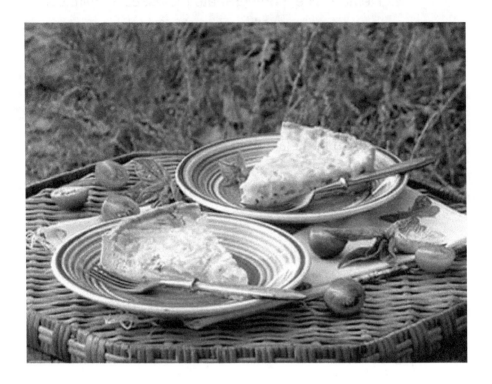

Preparation Time: 10 minutes

Cooking Time: 35 minutes

Yield: 8 slices

Ingredients

- 1 medium tomato (sliced into thin rounds)
- Extra-virgin olive oil
- 1 zucchini (sliced into rounds)
- 3 shallots (sliced into rounds)
- Salt and pepper

- 1 teaspoon sweet Spanish paprika
- ½ cup mozzarella (shredded)
- 2 tablespoons Parmesan (grated)
- 3 large eggs (beaten)
- ⅔ cup skim milk
- ¼ teaspoon baking powder
- ½ cup white whole wheat flour (sifted)
- ¼ cup fresh parsley

Directions

1. Start by preheating the oven to 350°F.
2. Place the sliced tomatoes on a paper towel and sprinkle with salt. Set aside and leave for a few minutes.
3. Meanwhile, in a large skillet, heat 2 tablespoons of extra-virgin olive oil over medium heat. Add zucchini and shallots. Season with salt, pepper, and ½ teaspoon of paprika. Sautee, stirring occasionally, until vegetables are tender.
4. Arrange the zucchini, shallots, and sliced tomatoes in a slightly oiled 9-inch pie dish. Sprinkle the Mozzarella and Parmesan evenly on top.
5. In a mixing bowl, combine eggs, remaining ½ teaspoon paprika, baking powder, fresh parsley, flour and milk; whisk together until smooth and pour into pie dish on top of the cheese mixture.

6. Bake in preheated oven for about 30 minutes until the egg mixture is set.
7. Remove from oven. Cool slightly before slicing.

Nutrition Facts

Per serving (1 slice) | Calories: 145 | Fat: 5.6g | Saturated Fat 1.9g | Carbohydrates: 16.5g | Sugar: 3.3g | Sodium: 252.2mg | Protein 8.4g

Potato Hash with Veggies and Poached Eggs

Preparation Time: 10 minutes

Cooking Time: 14 minutes

Yield: 4 servings

Ingredients

- Extra-virgin olive oil
- 1 yellow onion (chopped)
- 2 cloves of garlic (chopped)
- 2 russet potatoes (diced)
- Salt and pepper
- 1 cup canned chickpeas (drained and rinsed)
- 16 ounces of asparagus (remove the hard ends and chop into ¼-inch pieces)
- 1½ teaspoons ground allspice
- 1 teaspoon Za'atar
- 1 teaspoon dried oregano
- 1 teaspoon sweet paprika
- 1 teaspoon coriander
- Pinch of sugar
- 4 eggs
- 1 teaspoon White Vinegar
- 1 red onion (finely chopped)
- 2 Roma tomatoes (chopped)
- ½ cup crumbled feta cheese

- 1 cup fresh parsley (chopped)

Directions

1. Place a skillet over medium heat and add $1\frac{1}{2}$ tablespoons olive oil. Once the oil is heated, increase the heat to medium-high; add chopped onions, garlic, and potatoes. Sprinkle with salt and pepper to taste. Cook for 5-7 minutes, stirring frequently, until the potatoes are tender or golden crust, depending on your preferences.
2. Add the chickpeas, asparagus, more salt and pepper to taste, and the spices. Cook an additional 5-7 minutes. Reduce the heat to low to keep your potato hash warm. Stir occasionally.
3. Meanwhile, fill the saucepan about $\frac{2}{3}$ full of water and bring to a boil then reduce the heat to a steady simmer. Stir the 1 teaspoon vinegar into the water.
4. Carefully crack the eggs into a bowl. Use a spoon to swirl the simmering water, creating a gentle whirlpool.
5. Gently add the eggs to the middle of the whirlpool and cook them for 3 minutes. Using a slotted spoon, remove eggs from water and drain on a clean kitchen towel. Season with salt and pepper.
6. Remove the potato hash from the heat and transfer to plates. Add chopped red onions, tomatoes, feta, and parsley. Top with the poached eggs and serve.

Nutrition Facts

Per serving (¼ recipe) | Calories: 535 | Fat: 20.8g | Saturated Fat: 6g | Carbohydrates: 34.5g | Sugar: 6.9g | Sodium: 295.8g | Protein: 26.6g

Tomato Greek Salad with Cheese

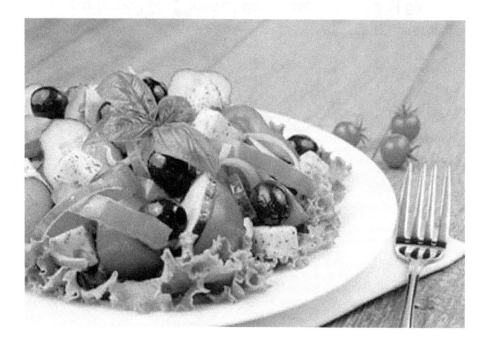

Preparation Time: 15 minutes

Cooking Time: 5 minutes

Yield: 4 servings

Ingredients

- 7 ounces Greek feta (halved)
- ½ cup Kalamata olives (pitted)
- 8.8 ounces red mini roma tomatoes (halved)
- 7 ounces yellow grape tomatoes (halved)
- 2 tablespoons extra-virgin olive oil
- 1 Lebanese cucumber (diced)

- ½ red onion (thinly sliced into rings)
- 1 green capsicum (diced)
- ¼ cup fresh oregano leaves
- 2 tablespoons lemon juice
- 1 garlic clove (crushed)

Directions

1. Dry feta cheese with a paper towel.
2. Place a non-stick frying pan over high heat and add 2 teaspoons olive oil. Once the oil is heated, add feta.
3. Cook one side of the feta cheese for 2 minutes until it turns golden.
4. Remove pan from heat. Stand feta in pan, without moving, for 10 minutes to cool slightly.
5. Meanwhile, in a large bowl, combine onions, olives, tomatoes, capsicum, cucumber, and half the oregano.
6. In a small bowl, mix garlic with lemon juice and oil. Sprinkle with salt and pepper to taste.
7. Pour dressing over the salad and toss to coat thoroughly.
8. Serve salad with feta cheese and garnish with oregano.

Nutrition Facts

Per serving (1 portion) | Calories: 316.9 | Total Fat: 24.2g | Saturated Fat: 9.6g | Carbohydrates: 8.6g | Sodium: 726mg | Fiber: 7g | Protein: 12.2g| Cholesterol: 34mg

Roasted Vegetables with Cheese and Olives

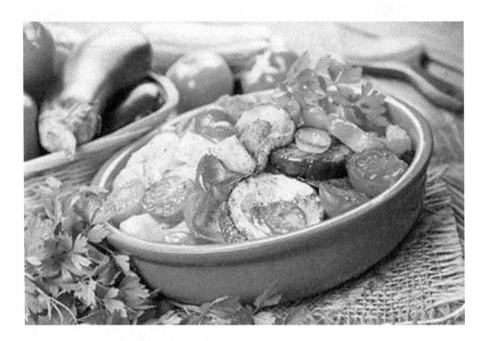

Preparation Time: 10 minutes

Cooking Time: 25 minutes

Yield: 4 servings

Ingredients

- 21 ounces packet frozen Mediterranean vegetable mix
- 1 lemon (cut into wedges)
- 1 red onion (cut into wedges)
- 3.5 ounces Greek feta (roughly crumbled)
- ⅓ cup Kalamata olives (pitted)
- 1 tablespoon red wine vinegar
- 2 tablespoons extra-virgin olive oil

- 1.7 ounces baby rocket

Directions

1. First, preheat the oven to 392°F.
2. Spread the frozen vegetables and lemon on the parchment lined roasting pan.
3. Add the onions, feta, and olives. Bake for 20 to 25 minutes until tender.
4. While waiting for the veggies, in a small bowl, whisk together vinegar and oil. Season with salt and pepper.
5. When the veggies are done, add baby rocket. Mix gently.
6. Transfer to a platter and serve with a generous amount of dressing.

Nutrition Facts

Per serving (1 portion) | Calories: 344 | Total Fat: 22.2g | Saturated Fat: 7.2g | Carbohydrates: 24.4g | Sodium: 889mg | Fiber: 4.5g | Protein: 8.9g | Cholesterol: 17mg

Roasted Olives

Preparation Time: 10 minutes

Cooking Time: 20 minutes

Yield: 3 servings

Ingredients

- 1 tablespoon extra-virgin olive oil
- ½ cup whole Kalamata olives
- 3 sprigs fresh oregano
- 3 small red chilies, split (stems attached)
- ½ cup whole green Sicilian olives
- 1 tablespoon drained capers
- 1 garlic clove (thinly sliced)
- Black pepper to taste

Directions

1. Start by preheating the oven to 392°F.
2. In a medium-sized bowl, place garlic, oregano, chilies, olives, and capers. Sprinkle with pepper. Mix to combine.
3. Transfer to an ovenproof dish. Drizzle with oil and then roast in the oven for 20 minutes or until olives are heated through. Stir once or twice while roasting.
4. Let it rest for 5 minutes and then serve.

Nutrition Facts

Per serving (1 portion) | Calories: 64 | Total Fat: 6.3g | Saturated Fat: 0.8g | Carbohydrates: 0.9g | Sodium: 298mg | Fiber: 0.9g | Protein: 0.5g

Pan Fried Chicken

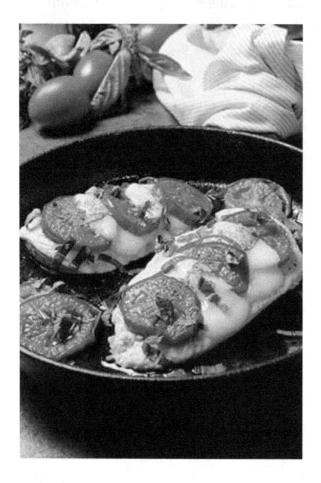

Preparation Time: 10 minutes

Cooking Time: 10 minutes

Yield: 4 servings

Ingredients

- Extra-virgin olive oil

- 1 pound of chicken breast (skinless, boneless and flattened with a kitchen mullet)
- Salt and black pepper
- 4 slices of fresh mozzarella cheese ($\frac{1}{2}$ inch in thickness)
- 3 tablespoons of Balsamic glaze
- 4 slices of ripe tomatoes
- 8 fresh basil leaves (leave 4 whole and slice the rest into ribbons)
- Basil pesto

Directions

1. Cut each breast in half horizontally then cut into thin pieces. Pound lightly using a meat mallet or rolling pin. Pat chicken dry with paper towel and season with salt and pepper to taste.
2. Heat up an indoor griddle or pan on high heat and drizzle with 1 tablespoon of extra-virgin olive oil.
3. Brown the chicken cutlets for about three minutes on each side, until they reach an internal temperature of 165°F. At the last couple minutes, add basil pesto and mozzarella slices on top of each chicken breast.
4. Remove from heat.
5. Add fresh basil leaves and tomato slices on top.
6. Glaze with balsamic vinegar on top and sprinkle fresh basil ribbons for the final touches.

Nutrition Facts

Per serving (1 portion) | Calories: 288 | Total Fat: 15.1g | Saturated Fat: 4.8g | Carbohydrates: 2.6g | Sugar: 1.2g | Sodium: 124.4mg | Protein: 34g

Rustic Greek Salad with Salmon

Preparation Time: 15 minutes

Cooking Time: 10 minutes

Yield: 4 servings

Ingredients

- 2 teaspoons fresh oregano leaves (finely chopped), plus extra leaves to serve
- ½ cup plain Greek-style yoghurt
- 3.5 ounces Greek feta (crumbled)
- 2 x 5.3 ounces packets hot-smoked salmon (skin discarded and flaked)
- 2 baby cos lettuce (quartered and washed)
- 7 ounces red grape tomatoes (halved)
- 1 Lebanese cucumber (thinly sliced)
- 1 small yellow capsicum (cut into ½-inch pieces)
- 1 red onion (thinly sliced into rings)
- ¾ cup pitted Kalamata olives
- 1 garlic clove (crushed)
- Lebanese bread rounds(torn)
- 1 tablespoon lemon juice

Directions

1. In a small bowl, mix chopped oregano, garlic, yogurt, juice, and 1 tablespoon warm water.

2. Sprinkle with salt and pepper to taste.
3. To prepare the salad, place the lettuce, cucumber, tomato, onion, olives, feta, capsicum, and salmon in a serving bowl.
4. Drizzle with a generous amount of yogurt dressing and top with oregano leaves.
5. Serve with bread and enjoy!

Nutrition Facts

Per serving (1 serving) | Calories: 546.8 | Total Fat: 20.7g | Saturated Fat: 7.9g | Carbohydrates: 51.6g | Sodium: 1369mg | Fiber: 7.6g | Protein: 33.9g | Cholesterol: 63mg

Mediterranean Lunch Recipes

Moroccan Meatballs

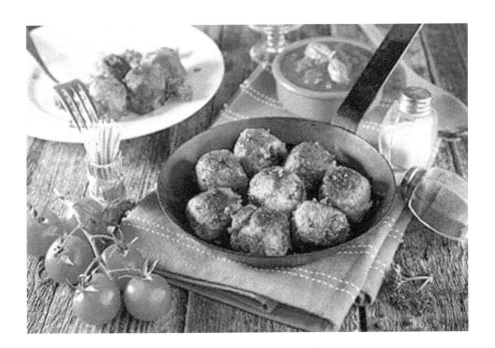

Preparation Time: 30 minutes

Cooking Time: 7 minutes

Yield: 30 meatballs

Ingredients

- 1 slice of bread (toasted and soaked in milk)
- 1¼ pounds lean ground beef
- 1 red onion (grated)
- 2 cloves of garlic (minced)

- Fresh cilantro (chopped)
- 3 teaspoons of Ras El Hanout spice blend*
- ½ teaspoon ground ginger
- ½ teaspoon cayenne
- Salt and pepper
- 3 tablespoons extra-virgin olive oil

Directions

1. Squeeze the excess milk out of the bread and place in a large bowl. Add the ground beef, onion, garlic, cilantro, Ras El Hanout, ginger, and cayenne. Season with salt and pepper to taste. Mix it all together.
2. Knead the mixture with your hands and portion into bite-sized balls. Line on a tray; cover and leave in a fridge for 30 minutes to make sure they maintain their form when fried.
3. Once ready, heat a skillet over medium heat. Drizzle meatballs with extra-virgin olive oil. Fry meatballs until cooked through, for 7 minutes, turning occasionally to make sure all sides are evenly cooked. Meatballs can be served with pita pockets or salads.

*Note: Ras el hanout is a classic spice mixture used in Moroccan cuisine. If you are unable to find it, here is a simple recipe for you to make your own.

1 part cumin + ½ part coriander + ½ part ginger powder + ½ part cayenne (or paprika if you like it milder).

Or use curry powder as substitute.

Nutrition Facts

Per serving (1 meatball) | Calories: 41 | Fat: 2g | Carbohydrates: 1.3g | Sugar: 0.4g | Sodium: 94.2 mg | Protein: 4.2 g

Mediterranean Socca Pizza

Preparation Time: 20 minutes

Cooking Time: 20 minutes

Yield: 2 servings

Ingredients

For Pizza Crust:

- 1¼ cup garbanzo bean flour
- 1¼ cup of cold water
- ¼ teaspoon sea salt
- ¼ teaspoon black pepper
- 2 tablespoons of olive oil or avocado oil
- 2 cloves of garlic (finely minced)
- 1 teaspoon of Onion powder (or other herbed seasoning or dried herbs)

For Pizza Toppings:

- 1 Roma tomato (sliced)
- ½ Avocado
- Gouda Cheese (sliced thinly)
- ¼ cup Tomato sauce
- 2 tablespoons chopped green onions
- Red pepper flakes (optional)

Directions

1. Begin by mixing flour, 2 tablespoons olive oil, water, and seasonings in a medium bowl. Whisk them together while making sure there are no lumps in the batter. Set aside for 15-20 minutes at room temperature.
2. As the base of your crust rests, preheat the oven to broil. Then, place a 10 to12-inchcast-iron skillet in the oven for 10 minutes. While the oven is preheating, slice and chop your vegetables.
3. After 10 minutes, take out your pan* and add 1 tablespoon of olive oil; swirl it around to grease the pan evenly. Slowly pour in your Socca batter, tilting the pan for an even distribution.
4. Turn the oven down to 425°F. Place the pan back in the oven and cook for 5-8 minutes. Check if the crust has set at 5 minutes, depending on how thick a batter you placed.
5. When the crust is cooked, take it out of the oven. Top the crust with tomato the sauce. Add sliced tomato, avocado, gouda slices, and green onions on top. You can also add more toppings, depending on your preferences.
6. Place the pan back in the oven for 10-15 minutes until cheese is melted and socca bread is crispy and brown outside. As an option, you can drizzle additional olive oil once your pizza is cooked.
7. Slice and serve.

*Note: Always use oven mitts or potholders when handling hot pots, pans, and baking trays so you don't burn yourself.

Nutrition Facts

Per serving (½ recipe) | Calories: 416 | Fat: 25g | Saturated Fat: 4.7g | Carbohydrates: 37g | Sugar: 7g | Sodium: 257mg | Fiber: 10g | Protein: 15g

Eggplant Wraps

Preparation Time: 15 minutes

Cooking Time: 35 minutes

Yield: 4 Eggplant Wraps

Ingredients

- 1 medium eggplant (evenly diced)
- 2 red bell peppers (diced)
- 1 medium white onion (finely chopped)
- 6 cloves of garlic (minced finely)
- 3 tablespoons of olive oil
- Salt and pepper
- 4 ounces of chevre cheese or any cheese you prefer
- 4 (8-inch each) flour tortillas
- 1 cup of sliced fresh basil leaves

Directions

1. After you've prepared all your ingredients, preheat your oven to 400°F.
2. Add eggplants, red bell peppers, onion, and garlic to the oven-safe skillet. Pour oil; sprinkle with salt and pepper to taste. Toss to coat. Place it in the oven to roast for 30 to 35 minutes.
3. Warm the chevre cheese or the cheese of your choice for around 15-20 seconds in a small microwavable bowl until it softens. Spread $\frac{1}{4}$ of the warmed cheese on the

tortilla, fill with some of the eggplant mix that was perfectly roasted in the oven, sprinkle with ¼ cup of basil, and then rollup.

4. They can be eaten right away or wrapped in plastic and refrigerated for later. They are perfect for a quick lunch or as appetizers when sliced.

Nutrition Facts

Per serving (1 eggplant wrap) | Calories: 431 | Fat: 23.4g | Saturated Fat: 8.9g | Carbohydrates: 43.8g | Sugar: 13.4g | Sodium: 491mg | Protein: 13.2g

Lemon and Greens Pasta

Preparation Time: 10 minutes

Cooking Time: 10 minutes

Yield: 4 servings

Ingredients

- 8 ounces of whole grain spaghetti (or any gluten-free pasta)
- 4 cloves of garlic (thinly sliced)
- 3 cups of greens (kale, Swiss chard, or spinach) (chopped)
- 1 small onion (thinly sliced)
- 3 cups of water
- ½ teaspoon fine sea salt
- ¼ teaspoon pepper
- Red pepper (crushed)
- 8 ounces marinated sun-dried tomatoes (chopped)
- 1 lemon (juiced and zested)
- Vegan parmesan (for toppings)

Directions

1. Begin by warming the olive oil from the jar of sundried tomatoes in a large pot over low-to medium heat. Add the garlic and onions and cook 3 minutes.

2. Then, add chopped greens (if using spinach, wait to add it later with the tomatoes), water, salt, and pepper and bring it to a boil.
3. Add pasta and stir until everything is completely drenched in boiling water. Lower the heat, cover, and let it cook for approximately 7 minutes until the water is absorbed.
4. Turn off the heat and drain the excess oils off the sun-dried tomatoes then place them in the pot (toss in the spinach now, if that's what you're using).
5. Add the crushed red pepper, lemon zest, and fresh lemon juice. Stir everything until the greens are wilted.
6. Divide into bowls evenly and top with parmesan cheese.

Nutrition Facts

Per serving (385g) | Calories: 274 | Total Fat: 15.4g | Saturated Fat: 2.1g | Carbohydrates: 33.3g | Sugar: 2g | Sodium: 528 mg | Fiber: 7.1g | Protein: 7.8g

Zucchini Noodles with Tangy Shrimp

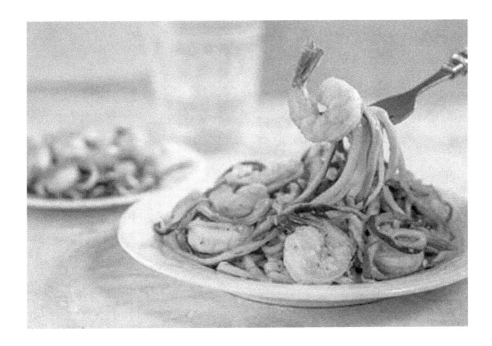

Preparation Time: 35 minutes

Cooking Time: 35 minutes

Yield: 4 servings

Ingredients

- 5-6 medium zucchini ($2\frac{1}{4}$-$2\frac{1}{2}$ pounds) (trimmed)
- 2 tablespoons butter
- 1 pound raw shrimp (peeled and deveined), tails left on if desired
- $\frac{1}{4}$ cup lemon juice
- 2 tablespoons extra-virgin olive oil,

- ½ teaspoon salt
- 2 cloves garlic (minced)
- 1 tablespoon cornstarch
- ⅓ cup white wine
- 3 tablespoons capers (rinsed)
- 1 cup low-sodium chicken broth
- 2 tablespoons fresh parsley (chopped)

Directions

1. Use a spiral vegetable slicer to cut zucchini lengthwise. This will produce long, thin strands that will be used as noodles. Make sure not to include the seeds.
2. Transfer the zucchini noodles to a colander and sprinkle with salt. Toss to distribute and leave colander over a mixing bowl or the sink to drain. Let sit for 20 to 30 minutes, giving an occasional squeeze.
3. In the meantime, melt butter with 1 tablespoon oil in a large skillet over medium-high heat. Add garlic and cook for 30 seconds, stirring constantly.
4. Add shrimp and cook for a minute until it changes color.
5. In a small bowl, combine broth with cornstarch. Add the cornstarch mixture to the shrimp, along with the lemon juice, capers, and wine.
6. Simmer and stir occasionally for 4 to 5 minutes until the shrimp is cooked. Remove from heat.
7. Using a large skillet, heat remaining tablespoon of oil over medium-high heat. Add zucchini noodles and cook, stirring and tossing them with tongs, for 2-3 minutes until slightly softened.

8. Serve the zucchini noodles with cooked shrimp and sauce. Garnish with parsley and serve!

Nutrition Facts

Per serving (1 cup zucchini and ¾ cup sauce) | Calories: 280 | Total Fat: 15g | Saturated Fat: 5g | Carbohydrates: 13g | Sodium: 516mg | Fiber: 3g | Protein: 24g | Cholesterol: 174mg | Sugars: 6g

Mediterranean Fish with Cherry Tomatoes and Olives

Preparation Time: 15 minutes

Cooking Time: 45 minutes

Yield: 4 servings

Ingredients

- 1 shallot (thinly sliced)
- 1 clove of garlic (thinly sliced)
- 2 pints of cherry tomatoes (halved)
- ¼ cup of extra-virgin olive oil + 2 tablespoons extra
- Salt
- 4 (6 ounce each)flounder or flat fish fillets
- ½ cup black olives (pitted)
- A handful of fresh Italian parsley, chives, and/or basil (chopped)

Directions

1. Preheat the oven to 400°F.
2. Place the shallot, garlic, and tomatoes on a parchment lined baking sheet and drizzle with ¼ cup of olive oil; season with 1 teaspoon salt. Mix everything together.
3. Roast the mixture in the oven until the tomatoes wrinkle and the juices are bubbling, for around 20 minutes.

4. Remove from the oven and stir the mixture. Place the fillet fish on top of the mixture in a single layer. Drizzle with 2 tablespoons of olive oil and season with 1 teaspoon salt. Arrange olives on top of the fish.
5. Place it back in the oven and cook until the fish turns flaky, about 10-15 minutes. Sprinkle the chopped herbs on top of a dish.
6. Serve.

Nutrition Facts

Per serving (1 portion) | Calories: 356 | Fat: 26.5g | Saturated Fat: 4.1g | Carbohydrates: 8.7g | Sugar: 4.6g | Sodium: 648mg | Fiber: 2.7g | Protein 23.4g

Roasted Citrus Branzino

Preparation Time: 20 minutes

Cooking Time: 1 hour

Yield: 4 servings

Ingredients

- 2 teaspoons of olive oil
- 8 ounces of pancetta (cut into ¼-inch dices)
- 2 whole branzino, about 1½ pounds each (scaled, gutted, and head removed)
- Salt and ground pepper
- 2 lemons (zested and thinly sliced)
- 1 medium fennel bulb, fronds coarsely chopped (about ¼ cup), bulb thinly sliced
- 2 tablespoons Fresh thyme (chopped)
- ½ cup dry white wine

Directions

1. Begin by placing an oven rack on the lowest half of the oven, preheating to 400°F.
2. Place a skillet over medium heat and add olive oil. Once the oil is heated, add the pancetta and cook, stirring occasionally, until it browns and crisps, about 8-10 minutes. Transfer pancetta to a paper towel lined plate; set aside.

3. Line a baking sheet with foil and spray with vegetable oil. Place the fish in the center of the baking sheet. Use a knife to cut slits about 2 inches apart across the top of the fish. They do not need to be super-deep – just enough to cut through the skin. Season with salt and pepper to taste.
4. Mix half the lemon zest, fennel fronds, and thyme in a small bowl. Fill the cavities of the fish with the lemon mixture and place thin slices of lemon and fennel on top. Scatter the cooked pancetta around the fish. Pour the wine over the fish.
5. Lay the second piece of foil on top of the fish and crimp the edges of both top and bottom pieces of foil together to make a large packet. Roast in the oven for 30 to 35 minutes until the fish is flaky.
6. Once cooked, let rest a few minutes before serving. To serve, transfer the fish to a plate and sprinkle with remaining lemon zest.

Nutrition Facts

Per serving (1 portion) | Calories: 467 | Fat: 15.5g | Saturated Fat: 5.8g | Carbohydrates: 7.1g | Sugar: 2.5g | Sodium: 615mg | Fiber: 2.6g | Protein 64.6g

Low Fat Stuffed Peppers with Rocket Salad

Preparation Time: 15 minutes

Cooking Time: 30 minutes

Yield: 4 servings

Ingredients

- 2 teaspoons balsamic vinegar
- ¼ cup Kalamata olives (pitted and chopped)
- 4 red bell peppers (halved and deseeded)
- 2 vine-ripened tomatoes (deseeded and finely chopped)
- 1 can (14 ounces) cannellini beans (rinsed and drained)
- 1 zucchini (finely chopped)
- 2 ounces of crumbled feta cheese
- 3 green shallots (thinly sliced)
- ¼ cup fresh parsley (chopped)
- 7 ounces grape tomatoes
- 3.5 ounces baby rocket
- 2 teaspoons lemon rind (finely grated)
- Salt and pepper to taste

Directions

1. Prepare the ingredients. Preheat the oven to 390°F. Line a baking tray with baking paper before placing the bell peppers cut side up. Cook around 10 minutes.

2. In a medium-sized bowl, combine feta cheese, olives, parsley, beans, chopped tomatoes, green shallots, zucchini, and lemon rind. Toss and season with salt and pepper to taste.
3. When the bell peppers have been roasted, make sure to drain any excess juices. Divide the filling among the roasted peppers and bake for another 15 to 20 minutes or until the peppers are softened and golden.
4. While waiting for the peppers, toss halved grape tomatoes in a medium bowl. Add vinegar. Toss until evenly coated.
5. Serve with the peppers.

Nutrition Facts

Per serving (1 portion) | Calories: 242.4 | Total Fat: 7g | Saturated Fat: 3g | Carbohydrates: 23 g | Sodium: 484mg | Fiber: 12g | Protein: 14g

Grilled Veggie Pasta

Preparation Time: 10 minutes

Cooking Time: 12-15 minutes

Yield: 4 servings

Ingredients

- 13.2 ounces dried large spiral pasta
- 2.8 ounces semi-dried tomatoes (roughly chopped)
- 5.3 ounces chargrilled eggplant (chopped)
- 14.5 ounce can crushed tomatoes
- 5.3 ounce marinated artichokes (cut into wedges)
- ⅓ cup basil pesto
- 2.8 feta-stuffed green olives (halved lengthways)
- 3.5 ounces chargrilled capsicum (chopped)
- Shredded fresh basil leaves as garnish

Directions

1. Cook pasta according to the packet directions.
2. Heat a saucepan over medium-high heat and add the crushed tomatoes. Cook the tomatoes for 2 minutes. Add the artichoke, semi-dried tomatoes, eggplant, and capsicum and cook another minute.
3. Drain pasta completely and make sure to reserve ¼ cup cooking water. Add the sauce with the pasta in a saucepan.

4. Then mix in the reserved cooking water and olives. Cook for a minute while continuously stirring until the sauce thickens.
5. Add pesto and garnish with basil leaves. Serve and enjoy!

Nutrition Facts

Per serving (1 portion) | Calories: 552 | Total Fat: 17.1g | Saturated Fat: 3g | Carbohydrates: 78.4g | Sodium: 856 mg | Fiber: 8.5g | Protein 17g | Cholesterol: 4mg

Mediterranean Shrimp

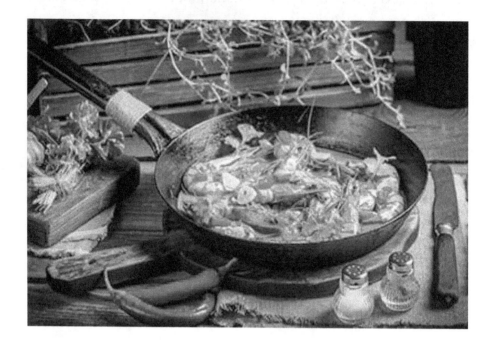

Preparation Time: 10 minutes

Cooking Time: 15 minutes

Yield: 4 servings

Ingredients

- 2 cups cooked rice (white or brown)
- 1¼ pounds of shrimp (peeled and deveined)
- 1 tablespoon all-purpose flour
- 2 teaspoons smoked paprika
- ½ teaspoon ground coriander
- ¼ teaspoon cayenne*

- ¼ teaspoon sugar
- 1 tablespoon butter
- 3 tablespoons extra-virgin olive oil
- 3 shallots (thinly sliced)
- 4 cloves of garlic (chopped)
- ½ green bell pepper(sliced)
- ½ yellow bell pepper(sliced)
- 1 cup diced tomato
- ⅓ chicken or vegetable broth
- 2 tablespoons dry white wine
- 2 tablespoons lemon juice
- ⅓ cup fresh parsley (chopped)
- ½ teaspoon each salt and pepper

Directions

1. In a large bowl, place flour, smoked paprika, salt, pepper, coriander, cayenne, and sugar. Add shrimp to bowl and toss until fully coated.
2. Heat a medium skillet over medium heat. Add butter and olive oil to the skillet and allow the butter to melt completely. Add your shallots and garlic; sauté for 2-3 minutes, stirring regularly until fragrant. Then add bell peppers and cook an additional 4 minutes, stirring occasionally.
3. Add the shrimp and cook 1-2 minutes. Add the tomatoes, broth, white wine, and lemon juice. Cook another 5 minutes until shrimps turn orange.

4. Serve with cooked rice and garnish with freshly chopped parsley.

*Note: For an extra kick, add one small sliced red chili pepper.

Nutrition Facts

Per serving (¼ recipe) | Calories: 281 | Fat: 13.5g | Saturated Fat: 2.7g | Carbohydrates: 10.2g | Sugar: 4.8g | Sodium: 244.6mg | Protein: 31.7g

Herb Salmon with Legume Salad

Preparation Time: 15 minutes

Cooking Time: 30 minutes

Yield: 4 servings

Ingredients

- 7 ounces green round beans (halved diagonally and blanched)
- 14 ounces frozen broad beans
- 5.2 ounces frozen peas (blanched)
- 5.2 ounces snow peas (halved diagonally and blanched)
- 1 tablespoon fresh rosemary (chopped)
- 4 (about 4.5 ounces each) salmon fillets
- 3.5 ounces baby spinach leaves
- 1.7 ounces snow pea sprouts
- 2 tablespoons balsamic vinegar
- Natural yoghurt
- 2 tablespoons lemon juice
- ¼ cup fresh mint leaves
- 1 tablespoon fresh chives (chopped)
- 1 tablespoon fresh thyme leaves
- 2 tablespoons extra virgin olive oil
- 3 teaspoons lemon rind (finely grated)

Directions

1. Pour boiling water over broad beans. Stand for two minutes then drain and refresh in iced water for 2 minutes.
2. Drain, peel, and transfer to a large bowl. Toss baby spinach, snow peas, peas, beans, snow pea sprouts, and mint with the broad beans.
3. On a plate, combine chives, thyme, rosemary, and lemon rind.
4. Season with salt and pepper to taste. Gently rub herb and citrus mixture into fish, spreading evenly.
5. Heat a large frying pot over medium heat and spray it with cooking oil.
6. Fry salmon for 2-3 minutes then turn over and fry another 2-3minutes or until cooked through.
7. Sprinkle oil and vinegar onto the salad and toss. Spoon the salad onto each of four serving plates and serve the salmon alongside it.
8. Drizzle the dish with lemon juice and serve with yoghurt.

Nutrition Facts

Per serving (1 portion) | Calories: 430 | Total Fat: 18g | Saturated Fat: 3.5g | Carbohydrates: 25g | Fiber: 12g | Protein: 44g

Mediterranean Baked Snapper

Preparation Time: 25 minutes

Cooking Time: 1 hour

Yield: 8 servings

Ingredients

- ⅔ cup extra-virgin olive oil
- 1 teaspoon caraway seeds
- ⅓ cup Kalamata olives
- ⅔ cup dry white wine
- 14 ounces cherry truss tomatoes
- 4 garlic cloves (crushed)
- 2 teaspoons ground coriander
- 1 teaspoon sweet paprika
- ⅔ cup fresh oregano leaves, plus extra to serve
- ⅔ cup fresh dill sprigs, plus extra to serve
- 2 teaspoons finely grated lemon rind
- 2.2 pounds red-skinned potatoes, cut into 0.4-inch slices
- 2 tablespoons lemon juice
- 3.3 pounds whole cleaned snapper
- 2 tablespoons drained capers, rinsed
- Lemon wedges, to serve

Directions

1. Preheat oven to 390°F.
2. In a large bowl, crush half the tomatoes that have been removed from the vine. Add lemon juice, garlic, wine, coriander, 1 tablespoon of oil, and paprika. Sprinkle with salt and pepper to taste.
3. Stir the ingredients gently. Add the potatoes and toss thoroughly.
4. Transfer the potato mixture on lightly greased baking tray and place in the oven for 30 minutes.
5. While waiting for the potatoes, place dill, caraway seeds, rind, oregano, and remaining oil in a food processor. Season with salt and pepper.
6. Process until finely chopped.
7. Slash the flesh of the fish 3-4 times on each side. Rub the dill mixture onto the fish, making sure the cavity and slits are well-coated. Put fish on top of the potato mixture and bake 15 minutes.
8. Add the capers, olives, and remaining tomatoes onto the tray and bake another 15 minutes until fish is cooked.
9. Sprinkle with herbs and garnish with lemon wedges. Serve hot.

Nutrition Facts

Per serving (1 portion) | Calories: 359.2 | Total Fat: 11.5g | Saturated Fat: 2.1g | Carbohydrates: 16.1g | Sodium: 351mg | Fiber: 4.8g | Protein: 42.3g | Cholesterol: 114mg

Gnocchi Salad

Preparation Time: 15 minutes

Cooking Time: 15 minutes

Yield: 4 servings

Ingredients

- 1 tablespoon red-wine vinegar
- 2 tablespoons extra-virgin olive oil
- 1 tablespoon fresh oregano (chopped), plus more for garnish
- 1 small onion (sliced)
- 1 (16-ounce) package gnocchi
- 4 large cloves garlic (thinly sliced)
- 1 (15-ounce) can chickpeas (rinsed)
- 1 (14-ounce) can no-salt-added diced tomatoes
- 1 small red bell pepper (diced)
- 8 pitted Kalamata olives (sliced)
- ¼ teaspoon ground pepper
- 1 (9-ounce) box frozen artichoke hearts (thawed and chopped)

Directions

1. Place a skillet over medium-high heat and add 1 tablespoon olive oil. Once the oil is heated, add gnocchi and cook 5 minutes, stirring often to prevent them from sticking together.

2. Transfer to a bowl, cover, and set aside.
3. Set the heat to medium and add the remaining tablespoon of oil. Add onions and sauté until brown for 2 to 3 minutes, stirring occasionally.
4. Add the bell peppers and cook another 3 minutes until they are crisp and tender. Add oregano and garlic, stirring from time to time for 30 seconds.
5. Stir in the artichokes, tomatoes, and chickpeas and cook until hot for around 3 minutes. Add pepper, vinegar, olives, and the gnocchi.
6. Garnish with oregano and serve.

Nutrition Facts

Per serving (1¾ cups) | Calories: 427 | Total Fat: 11g | Saturated Fat: 1g | Carbohydrates: 71g | Sodium: 615mg | Fiber: 10g | Protein: 12g | Sugars: 5g

Fish Fillets with Roast Tomatoes

Preparation Time: 5 minutes

Cooking Time: 15 minutes

Yield: 4 servings

Ingredients

- 4 (4-ounce) fresh or frozen skinless cod fillets ($\frac{3}{4}$- to 1-inch thick)
- 1 teaspoon fresh thyme (snipped)
- 2 teaspoons capers
- 3 cups cherry tomatoes
- $\frac{1}{4}$ teaspoon garlic powder
- 2 teaspoons fresh oregano (snipped)
- $\frac{1}{4}$ teaspoon black pepper
- 1 tablespoon olive oil
- $\frac{1}{2}$ teaspoon salt
- Nonstick cooking spray
- 2 cloves garlic (sliced)
- $\frac{1}{4}$ teaspoon paprika
- 2 tablespoons pitted ripe olives (sliced)
- Fresh oregano and/or thyme leaves

Directions

1. Thaw fish if frozen. Rinse and dry with paper towels.

2. Set oven to 450°F.
3. Combine oregano, salt, thyme, garlic powder, black pepper, and paprika in a small bowl. Generously coat both sides of the fillets with half the herb mixture.
4. Use foil to line a 15x10x1-inch baking pan and coat with cooking spray.
5. Arrange the fish on one side of the pan. Add the garlic and tomatoes on the other.
6. Mix the remaining oregano mixture with oil and drizzle over the tomatoes. Gently toss to coat tomatoes evenly.
7. Bake for about 8 to 12 minutes until the fish is flaky. Give the tomato mixture a quick stir about halfway through cooking. Once the tomatoes are cooked, add the olives and capers.
8. Transfer fish and roasted tomato mixture to a serving bowl.
9. Garnish with thyme or oregano leaves and serve.

Nutrition Facts

Per serving (1 cod fillet and ½ cup tomato mixture) | Calories: 157 | Total Fat: 5g | Saturated Fat: 1g | Carbohydrates: 7g | Sodium: 429 mg | Fiber: 2g | Protein: 22g | Cholesterol: 49mg | Sugar: 4g

Mediterranean Dinner Dishes

Chicken with Veggies and Lemon Vinaigrette

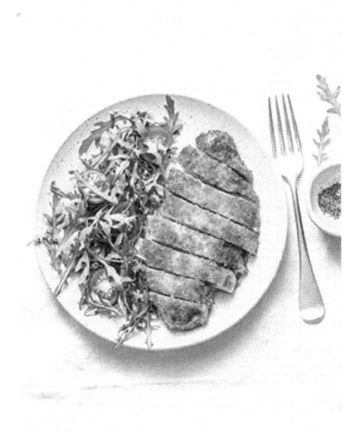

Preparation Time: 20 minutes

Cooking Time: 20 minutes

Yield: 4 servings

Ingredients

For Lemon Vinaigrette:

- ½ teaspoon lemon zest
- 1 tablespoon lemon juice
- ½ teaspoon honey
- 1 tablespoon feta cheese (crumbled)
- 1 tablespoon olive oil

For Chicken with Roasted Vegetables:

- 2 (8 ounce) skinless, chicken breast fillets (cut in half lengthwise)
- ¼ cup light mayonnaise
- 6 cloves garlic (minced)
- ½ cup panko bread crumbs
- 3 tablespoons grated Parmesan cheese
- ½ teaspoon kosher salt
- ½ teaspoon black pepper
- Nonstick olive oil cooking spray
- 2 cups 1-inch pieces asparagus
- 1½ cups sliced fresh cremini mushrooms
- 1½ cups grape tomatoes (halved)
- 1 tablespoon olive oil
- fresh dill

Directions

1. Prepare the vinaigrette: In a small bowl, combine lemon juice and zest with honey, feta cheese, and olive oil.
2. Prepare the vegetables and chicken: Begin by placing a 15x10-inch baking pan in preheated oven at 475°F.
3. Put the chicken breasts side by side on a cutting board and lay a piece of plastic wrap over them; pound with a flat meat mallet until they are about $\frac{1}{2}$-inch thick. Don't beat the chicken so much that it's falling apart.
4. In a medium bowl, combine the flattened chicken with 2 garlic cloves and mayonnaise. Stir gently until the chicken is well-coated.
5. In a flat dish, mix cheese, breadcrumbs, and $\frac{1}{4}$ teaspoon of salt and pepper. Press chicken onto the breading until evenly coated. Lightly coat the chicken with cooking spray.
6. Using a large bowl, combine oil, tomatoes, asparagus, mushrooms, 4 cloves of garlic, and $\frac{1}{4}$ teaspoon of salt and pepper.
7. Gently place chicken in one end of pan and place the vegetables on the other end. Roast in the oven for 18 to 20 minutes until vegetables are tender and chicken is done.
8. Sprinkle the lemon vinaigrette onto chicken and vegetables. Garnish with dill and serve.

Nutrition Facts

Per serving ($3\frac{1}{2}$ ounces of chicken and $\frac{1}{2}$ cup of vegetables) | Calories: 306 | Total Fat: 15g | Saturated Fat: 3g |

Carbohydrates: 12g | Sodium: 432mg | Fiber: 2g | Protein: 29g | Potassium: 616mg | Cholesterol: 90mg

Roasted Mushrooms

Preparation Time: 20 minutes

Cooking Time: 30 minutes

Yield: 4 servings

Ingredients

- 8 large flat mushrooms (stems removed)
- Olive oil spray
- 14 ounces fresh low-fat ricotta
- 1 large zucchini (coarsely grated and drained)
- 4 shallots (thinly sliced)
- 2 ounces (¼ cup) semi-dried tomatoes (finely chopped)
- 1 ounce Pitted Kalamata Olives (coarsely chopped)
- ¼ cup fresh basil leaves (chopped)
- 2 tablespoons pine nuts (toasted)
- 1 egg (lightly whisked)
- 3.5 ounces baby rocket leaves
- 4 slices sourdough bread (chargrilled)

Directions

1. Begin by preheating the oven to 392°F.
2. Spray mushrooms with oil and arrange on a lined baking tray.

3. In a medium-sized bowl, mix zucchini, shallots, ricotta, olive, tomato, basil, eggs, and pine nuts. Season with pepper.
4. Press mixture into mushrooms and cover with foil.
5. Bake 15 minutes and then remove the foil. Bake another 10 to 15 minutes until mushrooms are tender.
6. Serve hot with bread and rocket. Enjoy!

Nutrition Facts

Per serving (1 portion) | Calories: 331 | Total Fat: 15g | Saturated Fat: 5g | Carbohydrates: 22g | Sodium: 483.14mg | Fiber: 6g | Protein: 23g | Cholesterol: 104mg

Pan-fried Fish

Preparation Time: 10 minutes

Cooking Time: 15 minutes

Yield: 4 servings

Ingredients

- 7 ounces of cherry tomatoes (cut in half)
- 14 ounces green beans (topped)
- Sea salt flakes, to serve
- 2.2 ounces (⅓ cup) Kalamata olives
- 1 long fresh green chili (deseeded and thinly sliced)
- ¼ cup fresh continental parsley leaves
- 1 small red onion (halved and thinly sliced)
- 4 (about 5 ounces each) perch fillets
- ¼ cup olive oil
- 1½ tablespoons fresh lemon juice
- Steamed chat (baby coliban) potatoes, to serve
- Lemon wedges, to serve

Directions

1. Preheat oven to 430°F. On a baking tray, scatter the chili, onions, tomatoes, and olives. Drizzle with 2 tablespoons oil and stir. Cover the baking tray with aluminum foil and bake about 10 minutes until tomatoes are soft.

2. In the meantime, pour the remaining oil into a frying pan and put the pan over medium heat. Once the oil is heated, add the fish and cook 3 minutes per side or until fish is done when easily flaked with a fork.
3. In a saucepan, bring water to a boil and add the beans; cook for 3 to 4 minutes until tender. Drain the beans of excess water.
4. Add lemon juice, parsley, and beans to tomato mixture and stir.
5. Place the tomato mixture on individual serving plates and top with fish. Season with sea salt flakes. Serve with lemon wedges and potatoes.

Nutrition Facts

Per serving (1 portion) | Calories: 527.2 | Total Fat: 41g | Saturated Fat: 9g | Carbohydrates: 4g | Sodium: 369.96 mg | Fiber: 5g | Protein: 33g | Cholesterol: 116 mg

Carrot Salad

Preparation Time: 25 minutes

Cooking Time: 1 hour and 30 minutes

Yield: 8 servings

Ingredients

- 3.5 pounds large carrots (peeled and cut into 0.4 inch thick slices diagonally)
- 1 bunch mint (torn)
- 2 x 14-ounce cans chickpeas (rinsed and drained)
- ½ cup olive oil
- ⅓ cup fresh lemon juice
- 1½ teaspoons cumin seeds

Directions

1. First, preheat the oven to 375°F. Toss the carrot with oil in a large bowl.
2. Arrange half the carrots on a large roasting pan in a single layer and place in the oven for 20 minutes. Remove the pan from the oven, turn carrots, sprinkle with half the cumin seeds and return to the oven, and continue cooking for 20 minutes longer until carrots are soft and golden. Transfer to a large bowl.
3. Repeat with the rest of the carrots and cumin seeds.

4. Add the mint leaves, lemon juice, chickpeas, salt and pepper. Stir gently.
5. Serve and enjoy.

Nutrition Facts

Per serving (1 portion) | Calories: 262.9 | Total Fat: 16g | Saturated Fat: 2g | Carbohydrates: 20g | Sodium: 231.11 mg | Fiber: 11g | Protein: 6g

Grilled Salmon with Veggies

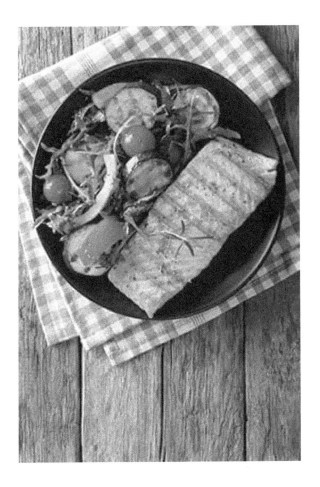

Preparation Time: 20 minutes

Cooking Time: 20 minutes

Yield: 4 servings

Ingredients

- 1¼ pounds salmon fillet (cut into 4 portions)

- 2 bell peppers(trimmed, halved and seeded)
- 1 medium zucchini (halved lengthwise)
- 1 medium red onion (cut into 1-inch wedges)
- ½ teaspoon salt
- ½ teaspoon ground pepper
- 1 tablespoon extra-virgin olive oil
- 1 lemon (cut into 4 wedges)
- ¼ cup fresh basil (thinly sliced)

Directions

1. Set grill to medium-high.
2. Take the peppers, onions, and zucchini and brush them with olive oil then sprinkle with ¼ teaspoon of salt. Season salmon with pepper and remaining salt.
3. Arrange the vegetables and salmon on the grill, skin-side down.
4. Cook the vegetables for 4 to 6 minutes per side, turning once or twice, until they are tender and have grill marks.
5. Grill the salmon for 8 to 10 minutes without turning until the fish is flaky.
6. Once cooked, let the vegetables cool then chop roughly and toss together in a large bowl.
7. Transfer the salmon and vegetables to individual plates, top with the basil, and serve with lime wedges.

Nutrition Facts

Per serving (1¼ cups of vegetables and a piece of salmon) | Calories: 281 | Total Fat: 13g | Saturated Fat: 2g | Carbohydrates: 11g | Sodium: 369mg | Fiber: 3g | Protein: 30g | Cholesterol: 66mg | Sugar: 6g

Crusted Salmon with Herbs and Nuts

Preparation Time: 10 minutes

Cooking Time: 15-20 minutes

Yield: 4 servings

Ingredients

- 1 (1 pound) skinless salmon fillet
- 1 clove garlic (minced)
- ¼ teaspoon lemon zest
- 2 teaspoons Dijon mustard
- 1 teaspoon lemon juice
- 3 tablespoons finely chopped walnuts
- ½ teaspoon honey
- ¼ teaspoon crushed red pepper
- 1 teaspoon fresh rosemary (chopped)
- 3 tablespoons panko breadcrumbs
- 1 teaspoon extra-virgin olive oil
- Olive oil cooking spray
- ½ teaspoon kosher salt

Directions

1. Preheat oven to 425°F.
2. In a small bowl, mix garlic, lemon zest, lemon juice, mustard, rosemary, salt, honey, and crushed red pepper. In another bowl, mix panko, oil, and walnuts.

3. Add the salmon fillets to a parchment paper-lined baking sheet. Top the fish with the mustard mixture and spread evenly with a spoon.
4. Sprinkle generously with the panko mixture and tap gently to make the breading stick. Coat lightly with cooking spray.
5. Transfer baking sheet to oven and bake approx. 8 to 12 minutes until flaky.
6. When the fish is done, carefully transfer to a serving plate.

Nutrition Facts

Per serving (3 ounces) | Calories: 222 | Total Fat: 12g | Saturated Fat: 2g | Carbohydrates: 4g | Sodium: 256 mg | Protein: 24g | Sugar: 1g | Cholesterol: 62mg

Greek Nacho Salad

Preparation Time: 15 minutes

Yield: 6 servings

Ingredients

- ⅓ cup prepared hummus
- 1 cup romaine lettuce (chopped)
- ¼ cup feta cheese (crumbled)
- 1 tablespoon lemon juice
- ¼ teaspoon ground pepper
- 2 tablespoons extra-virgin olive oil
- 3 cups whole-grain pita chips
- 1 tablespoon fresh oregano (minced)
- 2 tablespoons Kalamata olives (chopped)
- ½ cup grape tomatoes (quartered)
- 2 tablespoons red onion(minced)

Directions

1. Whip oil, lemon juice, pepper, and hummus in a small bowl.
2. Arrange pita chips in one layer on a serving platter.
3. Spread ¾ of the hummus mixture over the chips. Top with tomatoes, feta cheese, olives, red onions, lettuce, and a dollop of the remaining hummus.
4. Garnish with oregano and serve.

Nutrition Facts

Per serving (1 serving) | Calories: 159 | Total Fat: 10g | Saturated Fat: 2g | Carbohydrates: 13g | Sodium: 270mg | Fiber: 2g | Protein: 4g | Potassium: 116mg | Sugar: 2g | Cholesterol: 6mg

Pan Seared Chicken in Tomato Sauce

Preparation Time: 20 minutes

Cooking Time: 25 minutes

Yield: 4 servings

Ingredients

- 2 skinless chicken breasts (8 ounces each)
- ½ teaspoon salt
- ½ teaspoon ground pepper
- ¼ cup white whole-wheat flour
- 3 tablespoons olive oil
- ½ cup cherry tomatoes (halved)
- 2 tablespoons shallots (sliced)
- ¼ cup balsamic vinegar
- 1 cup low-sodium chicken broth
- 1 tablespoon garlic (minced)
- 1 tablespoon fennel seeds (toasted and lightly crushed)
- 1 tablespoon butter

Directions

1. Cut chicken breasts into halves lengthwise to make them thinner. Place on a cutting board and pound smooth with a meat mallet between 2 wax papers until

¼-inch thick. Season with ¼ teaspoon of pepper and salt.

2. Fill a shallow dish with flour and coat both sides of the chicken fillets. Tap off the excess.
3. Heat a large skillet over medium-high heat with 2 tablespoons of oil. Sear 2 pieces of chicken for 2 to 3 minutes per side, turning once until evenly browned.
4. Transfer to a serving plate and cover with cooking foil to keep warm. Repeat with the remaining chicken.
5. In the same pan, add a tablespoon of oil, shallots, and tomatoes.
6. Cook 1 to 2 minutes, stirring occasionally.
7. Add vinegar and bring to a boil, stirring and scraping up any browned bits from bottom of pan until the vinegar is reduced by half. Add fennel seeds, broth, garlic, and season with ¼ teaspoon pepper and salt.
8. Keep stirring until the sauce is reduced by half, 4 to 7 minutes. Remove from heat and add the butter.
9. Serve sauce on top of chicken.

Nutrition Facts

Per serving (3 ounces of chicken and 3 tablespoons of sauce) | Calories: 294 | Total Fat: 17g | Saturated Fat: 4g | Carbohydrates: 9g | Sodium: 371mg | Fiber: 1g | Protein: 25g | Sugar: 3g | Cholesterol: 70mg

Turkey Burgers with Cheese and Spinach

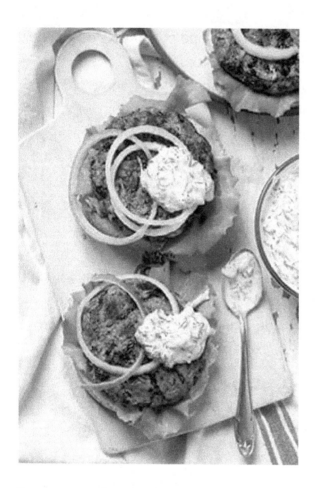

Preparation Time: 15 minutes

Cooking Time: 15 minutes

Yield: 4 servings

Ingredients

- 1 pound 93% lean ground turkey

- ½ teaspoon garlic powder
- 1 cup frozen chopped spinach, thawed
- ¼ teaspoon ground pepper
- ½ teaspoon dried oregano
- ½ cup crumbled Feta cheese
- 4 tablespoons Tzatziki
- 8 thick red onion rings (about ¼-inch)
- ¼ teaspoon salt
- 12 slices cucumber
- 4 small hamburger buns, split

Directions

1. Set grill to medium high.
2. Thaw and drain spinach. Squeeze between paper towels to remove all the liquid and combine with turkey, garlic powder, Feta cheese, oregano, salt and pepper. Mix well.
3. Using your hands, form four 4-inch thick patties.
4. Oil the grill rack. Place the patties on the grill for 4 to 6 minutes per side until it is cooked through or until the internal temperature reaches 165°F.
5. Arrange the patties on the burger buns and top each with a tablespoon of Tzatziki, 2 onion rings, and 3 cucumber slices. Serve hot and enjoy!

Nutrition Facts

Per serving (1 burger) | Calories: 375 | Total Fat: 17g | Saturated Fat: 6g | Carbohydrates: 28g | Sodium: 677mg | Fiber: 5g | Protein: 30g | Cholesterol: 103mg | Sugar: 5g

Caprese Chicken

Preparation Time: 25 minutes

Cooking Time: 25 minutes

Yield: 4 servings

Ingredients

- 2 boneless, skinless chicken breasts (8 ounces each)
- ½ teaspoon ground pepper, divided
- ½ teaspoon salt, divided
- ¼ cup prepared pesto
- 8 cups broccoli florets
- 1 medium tomato, sliced
- 2 tablespoons extra-virgin olive oil
- 3 ounces fresh mozzarella, halved and sliced

Directions

1. Coat a large rimmed baking pan with cooking spray and preheat the oven to 375°F.
2. Use paring knife to cut 6 crosswise ½-inch slits into top of each chicken breast, being careful not to cut all the way through to bottom of chicken.
3. Season with ¼ teaspoon of salt and pepper. Fill the cavities with alternating tomato and mozzarella slices.
4. Brush with pesto sauce and then transfer to one side of the baking sheet.

5. In a large bowl, toss oil, broccoli, and ¼ teaspoon of salt and pepper. You can also add any remaining tomatoes or cheese.
6. Place the broccoli mix onto the opposite side of the prepared baking sheet in a single layer.
7. Bake 25 minutes or until chicken is well-cooked and broccoli is tender.
8. Serve and enjoy!

Nutrition Facts

Per serving (½ chicken breast and 1 cup of vegetables) | Calories: 355 | Total Fat: 19g | Saturated Fat: 6g | Carbohydrates: 10g | Sodium: 634mg | Fiber: 4g | Protein: 38g | Sugar: 3g

Mediterranean Style Pork Chops

Preparation Time: 10 minutes

Cooking Time: 35 minutes

Yield: 4 servings

Ingredients

- 1 tablespoon finely snipped fresh rosemary or 1 teaspoon dried rosemary, crushed
- 4 boneless pork loin chops, cut ½ inch thick (1 to 1-½ pounds total)
- ¼ teaspoon freshly ground black pepper
- ¼ teaspoon salt
- 3 cloves garlic, minced

Directions

1. Set the oven to 425°F and line a shallow roasting pan with aluminum foil.
2. Season all sides of the chops with pepper and salt. Set aside.
3. In a small bowl, mix rosemary and garlic. Rub the mixture onto the chops, evenly coating all sides.
4. Arrange the chops on the rack in a shallow roasting pan and roast for 10 minutes.
5. Lower the temperature to 350°F and roast for another 25 minutes until juices run clear. Serve hot.

Nutrition Facts

Per serving (1 pork chop) | Calories: 161 | Total Fat: 5g |
Saturated Fat: 2g | Carbohydrates: 1g | Sodium: 192mg |
Cholesterol: 62mg | Protein: 25g

Penne with Tomato Sauce and Greens

Preparation Time: 10 minutes

Cooking Time: 15 minutes

Yield: 4 servings

Ingredients

- 12.3 ounces of Penne Rigati pasta
- 3.5 ounces of semi-dried tomatoes with mixed basil
- 24 ounces of tomato sauce
- 9.8 ounces ready to use char grilled mixed vegetables
- 3.5 ounces mild salami (thinly sliced)
- 9.7 ounces of marinated artichokes (drained and halved)
- ½ cup basil (finely shredded)
- ½ cup (2.1 ounce) Mediterranean mixed olives (pitted and thinly sliced)
- Parmesan,(finely grated), to serve

Directions

1. In a large saucepan, cook the pasta as instructed on the packet. Drain well afterwards.
2. Place a large saucepan over medium heat. Add the salami slices and cook until crisp, about 1 minute per side. As the slices are done, transfer them to a plate.

3. Then, add olives, vegetables, sauce, artichokes, and tomatoes to the pan and bring to a gentle simmer. Cook 5 minutes.
4. Pour the tomato mixture on top of the pasta and toss gently to combine.
5. Divide among the serving bowls, sprinkle with salami, and garnish with basil.
6. Add grated Parmesan cheese on top. Serve hot.

Nutrition Facts

Per serving (1 portion) | Calories: 640.5 | Total Fat: 25g | Saturated Fat: 5g | Carbohydrates: 82g | Protein: 22g

Eggplant Surprise

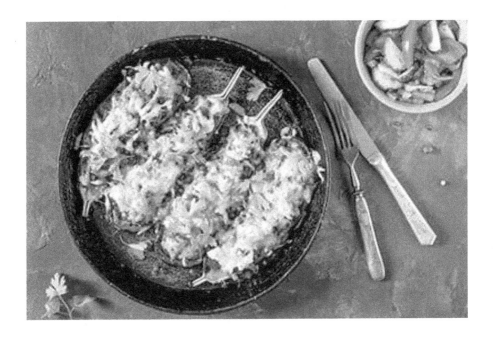

Preparation Time: 35 minutes

Cooking Time: 1 hour

Yield: 4 servings

Ingredients

- 2 small eggplants (12 ounces each)
- 2 tablespoons extra-virgin olive oil plus ¼ cup, divided
- 2 cloves garlic (chopped)
- ¼ teaspoon salt
- ½ teaspoon ground pepper
- ½ cup Parmesan cheese (finely grated)

- 1¼ cups fresh breadcrumbs
- 1 large egg (lightly beaten)
- ⅓ cup fresh parsley (chopped)
- 1 teaspoon capers (rinsed)
- 1¼ cups no-salt-added tomato sauce, divided
- 4 large basil leaves

Directions

1. While preparing the ingredients, preheat the oven to 375°F.
2. Cut the eggplant in half lengthwise with a large knife.
3. Trim the sides so the eggplant will lay flat. Hollow out inside of eggplant, leaving a sturdy shell for stuffing; set aside the shells. Roughly chop scooped-out eggplant flesh.
4. Place a medium saucepan with 2 tablespoons of oil over medium heat.
5. Add the chopped eggplant and cook 2 to 3 minutes until softened. Add garlic and cook 3 to 5 minutes.
6. Place in a bowl and season with ¼ teaspoon of pepper and salt.
7. Heat the remaining oil in a large skillet over medium heat. Sprinkle eggplant shells with pepper and 2 tablespoons of Parmesan cheese.
8. Cook in hot oil, turning once, 5 to 8 minutes until it turns golden brown. Transfer and let drain on plate covered with paper towels.

9. Place the breadcrumbs in a bowl of water and squeeze out the excess.
10. Transfer to a bowl with the eggplant flesh and add ¼ cup Parmesan, parsley, capers, and an egg.
11. Spoon the filling evenly into the shells.
12. Pour 1 cup of tomato sauce into an oven proof dish big enough to fit the eggplant in one layer.
13. Transfer the stuffed eggplant to the dish. Top each eggplant half with remaining tomato sauce, spreading evenly with a spoon. Garnish with basil and sprinkle 2 tablespoons of Parmesan.
14. Bake until the internal temperature reaches 160-165°F, about 25 minutes. Serve hot and enjoy!

Nutrition Facts

Per serving (½ eggplant) | Calories: 324 | Total Fat: 21g | Saturated Fat: 4g | Carbohydrates: 27g | Sodium: 470mg | Fiber: 7g | Protein: 9g | Cholesterol: 55mg | Sugar: 9g

Passata Infused Baked Fish

Preparation Time: 15 minutes

Cooking Time: 25 minutes

Yield: 4 servings

Ingredients

- 2 white fish fillets
- ⅓ cup fresh oregano leaves
- Olive oil spray
- 1½ cups passata (tomato pasta sauce)
- 1 cup couscous
- 1½ tablespoons olive oil
- ¼ cup black olive tapenade

Directions

1. Preheat oven to 356°F. Spray a baking pan with olive oil.
2. Transfer fish to prepared dish and spread tapenade evenly over the fish fillets.
3. Pour the passata and season with pepper to taste. Top each fish with oregano and drizzle with a tablespoon of olive oil.
4. Bake in the oven for 20-25 minutes until fish is flaky.
5. Pour 1 cup boiling water over one cup couscous. Add remaining oil and stir. Cover with a plate or plastic wrap

and set aside until the water is absorbed, about 10 minutes. Fluff with a fork.

6. Cut each fish fillet in half. To serve, spoon the couscous onto a serving plate and lay the fish fillet on top.

7. Drizzle with sauce and garnish with oregano.

Nutrition Facts

Per serving (1 portion) | Calories: 434 | Total Fat: 15g | Saturated Fat: 3g | Carbohydrates: 38g | Sodium: 55.05mg | Fiber: 4g | Protein: 34g | Cholesterol: 94mg | Sugar: 4g

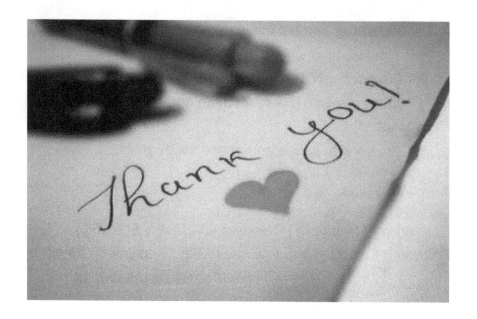

If you enjoyed this book or received value from it in any way, then I'd like to ask you for a favor: would you be kind enough to leave a review for this book on Amazon? It'd be greatly appreciated!

https://www.amazon.com/dp/B07Y41JJXG

Other books by Stephanie N. Collins You can find here

http://dexlerbooks.com/stephanie-n-collins